Praise for

ECSTASY *is* NECESSARY

"Barbara Carrellas is a brilliant writer. To Barbara, being sexual is as normal and comfortable as breathing, and she would like all of us to feel this way."

— **Louise Hay,** author of *Empowering Women* and *You Can Heal Your Life*

"If you long for connection to sacred joy, to the extraordinary, and to the healing power of full aliveness, then you'll love this book."

— **Cheryl Richardson**, author of *You Can Create an Exceptional Life*

"Ecstasy Is Necessary is destined to be a classic. Simply reading it is an ecstatic experience."

— **Denise Linn**, author of *Secrets and Mysteries: The Glory and Pleasure of Being a Woman*

"One of THE most brilliant books written on sex and relationships."

— **Mona Lisa Schulz, M.D., Ph.D.**, author of *The Intuitive Advisor*

"Barbara Carrellas is a true visionary. This book will give you the tools to create a bolder, more authentic, and satisfying sex life, but it goes much deeper: it's a road map for living a fuller, more conscious, and joyful life."

—**Tristan Taormino**, author of *Opening Up: A Guide to Creating and Sustaining Open Relationships*

"The exact book we need for these troubled, and troubling, times. Cultivating ecstasy as a spiritual practice, far from being selfish or shallow, allows us to live more fully in the world, with energy and love to spare, and share. More, please!"

— **Nina Hartley**, author of *Nina Hartley's Guide to Total Sex*

"Barbara Carrellas is the world's best ecstasy coach, and this book may be the best investment you'll ever make."

— **Annie Sprinkle, Ph.D.**, sex educator, ecosexologist, artist

ECSTASY *is* NECESSARY

Also by Barbara Carrellas

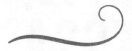

Luxurious Loving: *Tantric Inspirations for Passion and Pleasure*

Urban Tantra: *Sacred Sex for the Twenty-First Century*

ECSTASY *is* NECESSARY

a practical guide

barbara carrellas

HAY HOUSE, INC.
Carlsbad, California • New York City
London • Sydney • Johannesburg
Vancouver • Hong Kong • New Delhi

Published and distributed in the United States by: Hay House, Inc.: www.hayhouse.com® • *Published and distributed in Australia by:* Hay House Australia Pty. Ltd.: www.hayhouse.com.au • *Published and distributed in the United Kingdom by:* Hay House UK, Ltd.: www.hayhouse. co.uk • *Published and distributed in the Republic of South Africa by:* Hay House SA (Pty), Ltd.: www.hayhouse.co.za • *Distributed in Canada by:* Raincoast: www.raincoast.com • *Published in India by:* Hay House Publishers India: www.hayhouse.co.in

Cover design: Kate Basart/Union Pageworks
Cover photo: Joel Kubicki, Jr.
Interior design: Jenny Richards

Library of Congress Cataloging-in-Publication Data

Carrellas, Barbara.
  Ecstasy is necessary : a practical guide / Barbara Carrellas. -- 1st ed.
      p. cm.
  ISBN 978-1-4019-2847-6 (pbk. : alk. paper) 1. Sex. 2. Sex (Psychology) 3. Ecstasy. 4. Sexual excitement. I. Title.
  HQ23.C367 2012
  306.77--dc23   2011046412

Tradepaper ISBN: 978-1-4019-2847-6
Digital ISBN: 978-1-4019-3109-4

15   14   13   12   4   3   2   1
1st edition, March 2012

Printed in the United States of America

For Anne Francis
(1930–2011)

and

Chester Mainard
(1953–2007)

My voices from home.

CONTENTS

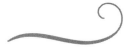

A Note about Pronouns

With this book, I'm going to revive an old linguistic tradition.

My books, like all of my work, are for people of all sexual preferences and all forms of gender expression, including people whose identity is something other than male or female. As such, I like to write with gender-neutral pronouns. However, English is sadly lacking in such pronouns. In recent years clever people have come up with alternatives to the use of "he" as the pronoun that applies to all genders. But words like "ze" and "hir" have not caught on in popular usage and a vast number of people find the use of these new pronouns distracting.

I found my personal solution to this dilemma in the history of the English language. Did you know that prior to 1745 there was an accepted and commonly used universal pronoun? The person who changed all that was Anne Fisher, an 18th-century British schoolmistress and the first woman to write an English grammar book. In 1745 Anne wrote the hugely popular "A New Grammar" in which she decreed that the pronoun "he" should apply to both sexes. For centuries before that, the universal pronoun had been "they." Writers as far back as Chaucer used it for masculine and feminine, singular and plural. So did Byron, Austen, Thackeray, Eliot, Dickens, Trollope, and more.

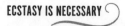

Well, I say if it's good enough for Chaucer it's good enough for me. So throughout this book I will use "they" whenever gender or plurality is unimportant. In doing so I hope it helps everyone to feel included in the discussion and that it inspires you to think outside of traditional sex and gender binaries.

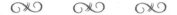

PRELUDE

This Is Your Brain on Science, or Ecstasy Meets Terror in the Lab

If a doctor had suggested I voluntarily insert my severely claustro-phobic self into an fMRI machine I simply would have said no. "It isn't worth it," I would've insisted. "Not for anything short of an operable brain tumor." That may sound dramatic but it's true. I am so severely claustrophobic I will change airline reservations rather than risk a middle or window seat.

So what was I doing in this medical facility, staring at a huge white machine with a terrifyingly tiny opening, about to undergo a brain scan for no good life-threatening reason? That's just what I asked myself as I lay on the cool laboratory floor in Newark, New Jersey. I was taking deep breaths, hoping my heart would soon stop racing. The mere sight of the fMRI machine had triggered an attack of supraventricular tachycardia, sending my heart into a

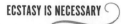

fight-or-flight reaction at nearly 200 beats per minute. Why had I even considered saying yes to this scan?

I was here because it *wasn't* a medical professional who asked me to do this brain scan. It was an orgasm researcher—an orgasm researcher and a documentary filmmaker. Together, this unlikely duo had made me an offer I simply couldn't refuse: the opportunity to find a scientific explanation for an erotic experience I could not otherwise explain.

It all began a month earlier when I received a call from an associate producer for a production company making a new series for the Discovery Channel. They wanted to do a short documentary on someone who could have an orgasm by "thinking off." At first I was not sure what they meant. I had been having orgasms without genital stimulation for years, but my technique was not entirely mental. More important than the visualization that went on in my head, was the conscious rhythmic breathing that carried me into my prolonged orgasmic states. Did they mean they were looking for people who could have an orgasm just by fantasizing? I certainly knew such people existed, but I was not one of them. No, the associate producer said, she was looking for people who could simply have an orgasm without any form of genital stimulation. I had been suggested to her by my friend and colleague, orgasm researcher Nan Wise. A Ph.D. candidate in Rutgers University's neuroscience department, she was working with Dr. Barry Komisaruk, one of a very few people of science doing research on what happens in the brain during orgasm.

I had known that Nan had been assisting Barry in his research into brain function during genitally produced orgasms. They scanned the brains of women as they pleasured themselves into orgasms in the lab. I certainly was not the only person I knew who could have a breath and energy orgasm, but I was certainly one of the people most passionately interested in them. I was fascinated by this study and longed to participate, but I had never volunteered because of my claustrophobia.

I first learned how to have a breath and energy orgasm in the late 1980s during the AIDS crisis. I was working in the Broadway theatre as a general manager. During those terrible times I had gone to the New York Healing Circle looking for emotional and spiritual support. By the late 1980s we were approaching the darkest of times. The theatre industry, with its disproportionately high percentage of gay men, was one of the communities particularly devastated by the epidemic. Some weeks I lost up to four friends, family members, or colleagues to AIDS. I arrived at the New York Healing Circle with an urgent need for help in dealing with the unrelenting and overwhelming grief I felt. In those days it was not uncommon to be in the hospital with one dying friend, only to learn that another had just passed away across town. People were dying so fast we could not mourn them properly. I wanted answers to those big questions we ask in times of tragedy. Questions like, "Is there a God?" and "If there is a God, how could they let this happen to us?"

The Healing Circle's big group meeting was in a high school auditorium on West 17th Street. Within my first hour I knew I had come to the right place. The circle was founded on the principles of self-love and positive thinking popularized by Louise Hay. Louise's weekly group in Los Angeles, the Hayride, was providing similar support to hundreds in the AIDS community on the West Coast. The love, comfort, encouragement, friendship, and relief in these groups was so authentic and uplifting that you left meetings feeling like you could walk on water. Within the first couple of meetings, the urgent needs that had brought me there were being met extremely well and I discovered a more compelling need—the need to help others.

Gay men had been at the forefront of the sexual revolution. They had taken the exploration and expression of sex to unparalleled heights and depths. And now all that was over. The sexual freedom that we had celebrated with such enthusiasm and abandonment in the '70s was now proclaimed to be the weapon of our destruction. We'd begun to practice the safest sex we possibly could—those of us who were having sex at all, that is. Some people in our community were so sick or so terrified that they stopped having sex. The rest of us wrapped ourselves in latex and hoped for the best. It was a precarious situation. I knew that people could not be scared into abstinence and safer sex forever. We had to find ways to have sex that would be spiritually nourishing, emotionally healing, and physically safe—and as ecstatic as it had been in the drug-enhanced, all-night mega-parties of the pre-AIDS era. At the Healing Circle I met two erotic pioneers, Joseph Kramer and Annie Sprinkle. They, too, were searching for this new way to be sexual. We enthusiastically joined forces. We became dearest friends, colleagues, and family.

We began our search in the East. Joseph had already been studying the principles of Taoist sexuality and had begun to combine them with massage and rebirthing. He was developing an erotic massage technique that was well on its way to becoming one of the paths to spiritually enlightening, healing, and hot sex. Annie, a well-known porn star, was turning her focus toward feminist erotic art and sexual healing. Annie and I began to study Tantra. In these Eastern spiritual practices, sex is seen not so much as an action one performs, but rather as an energy one allows. And nothing demonstrated moving energy into ecstasy like breath and energy orgasms.

A woman named Jwala facilitated the small workshop in which I had my first breath and energy orgasm. Jwala, whose name means Love Fire, would soon become my first Tantric teacher. I met her the way I met a lot of my teachers in that period—she had come to the Healing Circle as a guest speaker. Jwala was the ultimate hippie. She had no permanent home. She spent a great deal of time studying with her gurus in India. She was not like any spiritual seeker I had ever met. She was as sexual as she was mystical. Although in her that combination seemed natural and easy, I was initially skeptical. Something deep in my ex-Catholic background and career-driven New York personality bristled at her intense dedication to freedom, sexuality, and spirituality. I was envious of how happy she seemed. But Jwala was generously willing to teach me everything she knew, and the first was how to have a breath and energy orgasm.

We all sat in a circle on the floor as Jwala explained how the technique worked. "With each breath," she said, "imagine filling up each of your chakras—the seven major energy centers of the body—with energy." To demonstrate, Jwala lay on her back in the center of the circle and began to breathe. We watched her use her breath and imagination to pull energy from the earth into her body. She began with the first chakra (perineum), and moved up, chakra by chakra. Within a few minutes she was laughing and vibrating and writhing around on the floor. It was one of the juiciest and most joyous orgasms I had ever seen. And then it was our turn.

Jwala offered instructions in the form of a guided meditation. It wasn't sexual at all and at first I didn't feel anything. But I heard Jwala say, "Don't worry, just keep breathing," so I did. I imagined pulling energy up, chakra by chakra. By the time the energy reached my heart, I felt a tingling in my arms that started to spread into my chest and down my legs. I began to giggle. I felt like I'd been picked up by a huge wave that got taller and stronger with each breath. I discovered that all I had to do to stay on the wave was keep breathing. Jwala was still guiding us up the chakras but I was in freestyle. I laughed hysterically. I cried in big gulping sobs. I tingled all over. It felt like lightning bolts were shooting out my fingers. I felt like I was being animated by the gods. And it went on and on and on.

How could I not have known this existed? Why didn't *everyone* know how to do this? This ecstasy is what I imagined that sex could be—but seldom, if ever, was. And, oddly enough, this breath and energy orgasm had happened in every nook and cranny of my body *except* my genitals.

This ecstatic experience went far beyond pleasure. It was a profoundly transformative event that took me through all my emotions (including a few I hadn't met before). It was like bodysurfing in a whirlpool at the convergence of rivers named Emotion, Intuition, Mysticism, and Sex.

I was hooked. Breath and energy orgasms became the foundation of my personal erotic practice and the cornerstone on which I later built a career as a workshop facilitator and author.

And now here I was at a medical lab in Newark. After 20 years and countless breath and energy orgasms, I was about to find the answer to the questions I asked myself and had been asked by hundreds of workshop participants: Is this really an orgasm? Had I been fooling myself all these years? Was I simply hyperventilating? Or perhaps just throwing myself into breath-induced seizures? Did the brain know the difference between genital orgasms and these ecstatic, visionary, transcendental experiences that felt like full-body orgasms?

I arrived at the office of Dr. Barry Komisaruk at 9:30 A.M., accompanied by my friend Sarah Sloane. Sarah had answered my desperate plea for a piercer when I was told that the jewelry in all 18 of my body piercings would have to be removed for this scan. Some of the jewelry in these piercings had not been removed for 20 years and six pieces were impossible to remove or replace without professional help. But Sarah's presence this morning was about more than her piercing skills. I had not been *asked* to remove the jewelry, I had been *ordered* to. I do not respond well to orders. In addition to my apprehension about my claustrophobia, I now felt bullied, angry, and vulnerable about my piercings. I had done previous rituals with Sarah and she had always made me feel safe. She could be nurturing and supportive; she could also be fierce and protective. I would need all of her skills to get through today.

I'd learned that fMRI stands for functional magnetic resonance imaging. An fMRI machine is a big, expensive piece of medical equipment that generates high magnetic fields (hence the removal of metal jewelry) for the purpose of tracking brain activity. To be scanned in an fMRI machine, you lie on a horizontal stretcher-like platform that slides into the narrow cylindrical tunnel of the machine. When you're fully inserted into the machine, you are completely encircled to just below your waist.

An fMRI magnetically scans the patient from all sides. FMRIs reveal the brain's structure and its activity. It works like this: Active neurons in the brain consume more blood than inactive neurons. Therefore, more blood flows to particular areas of the brain when they are active. The hemoglobin in red blood cells is an "oxygen-storage molecule" which is capable of absorbing and releasing oxygen multiple times. The hemoglobin is oxygenated with air from the lungs and deoxygenated when it delivers the oxygen to the cells. Oxygenated and deoxygenated hemoglobin have different magnetic properties. Oxygenated hemoglobin is diamagnetic, which means that it slightly repels a magnetic field. Deoxygenated hemoglobin is paramagnetic, meaning that the application of an external magnetic field causes it to become slightly magnetic. The fMRI machine picks up the slightly magnetic quality of the deoxygenated hemoglobin in the active neural areas and delivers those results in a manner that allows researchers to study brain activity.

For an accurate scan the patient must lie very still. But how, I thought, could I have an orgasm without moving? I had practiced at home for a week, keeping my head braced between two stacks of pillows while I breathed myself to orgasm. I was reasonably convinced that I could do it without moving too much. But to get the scan, not moving very much was not enough. My head could not move *at all*. Dr. Barry explained that he was going to create a kind of plastic mesh helmet that could be placed around my head to hold it perfectly still. Hannibal Lecter came to mind. This was getting too freaky—even for me. I took slow, deep breaths. Dr. Barry asked if I was comfortable. Sarah looked like she'd punch someone if I said no. I found this reassuring.

Helmet completed, we now had to go to a nearby facility that actually had an fMRI machine. FMRI machines are expensive. You can't just ring up your local big-box store and order one because you need it for your science experiment that day. We had a precious couple of hours reserved in which to do this experiment. The clock had already started ticking when I took my first look at the terrifyingly tiny opening into which they intended to slide my helmeted body. I went into supraventricular tachycardia.

I tried to force myself to relax, which was, predictably, futile. I prayed, meditated, and pleaded for inner guidance to tell me if I should leave the lab immediately or hang in there until the tachycardia broke. All the while, Sarah alternated between trying to calm me in one room and the equally nervous television producers and orgasm researchers in the other.

Finally, the lead producer came into the room where I was lying on the floor. There was no more time left to decide. He told me that I did not have to do the scan if I felt I couldn't. They had worked out an alternative way to do the segment. I listened. I considered his offer. But the alternative would, of course, lack the definitive proof about *my* breath and energy orgasms. By this time, although the attack was not entirely over, I knew my heart was not going to explode. I could finally feel my intuition speak louder than my fear: "You can do this. The breath and energy orgasm is the way out of the panic you're feeling."

The television producers had been utterly respectful. They had not filmed a minute of my panic. I asked them to leave the cameras off for another minute while I got into the fMRI machine. With barely concealed relief and apprehension, they agreed. Dr. Barry and Nan put the plastic mesh helmet on my head and clamped it into a round steel frame attached to the platform bed of the fMRI machine. I felt like some helpless victim in a mid-1970s British horror film. Dr. Barry asked if I was ready.

"One more thing," I said. "Could you please put this blindfold over my eyes?" Dr. Barry looked surprised but agreeable as he taped the blindfold over the steel frame and the helmet.

Ahh. Better. Blindfolded, I could pretend that this was just an extremely kinky sex scene instead of medical torture. The most important reason for the blindfold was that my eyes often flutter open during a breath and energy orgasm. I knew that if my eyes opened and I could see that I was in this tiny tunnel, I would absolutely lose it. I had visions of bursting though the steel walls of the fMRI machine with my superhuman strength.

Then, one final thing—earplugs. I had only been concerned about the tiny enclosed space, but everyone I talked to about fMRIs warned me about the noise. Everyone was right. The clank, bang, slam, rumble is deafening. Good thing I am a longtime fan of loud, strange music. The earplugs reduced the cacophony enough so I could let it play in the background like an experimental score for some science-fiction movie.

At last they slid me into the fMRI machine. At first it was quiet. Before they could do the actual scan, they had to take still pictures of my brain. These still images would act as the canvas across which the brain activity would be shown. So I lay still in that tightly confining space as they fussed, adjusted, and calibrated. Luckily, I knew a way to cope. As a small child, I had learned to simply leave my body when conditions in my house were too claustrophobic and scary. So I drifted over to a corner of the lab, up near the ceiling, and waited for Nan, Dr. Barry, and the technician to finish. When they were ready for me to "think off," I slipped back into my body. I focused on my breath. I imagined erotic energy flowing in through the top of my head and the soles of my feet. I dropped an imaginary root down from my genitals all the way into the center of the earth. I imagined hot red erotic energy flowing in from below and bright hot sun pouring in from above.

Within moments I was traveling on one of the long journeys I'd come to associate with this kind of orgasm. It's rather like a magic carpet ride. I never know quite where in the cosmos I'll wind up, but I know it's someplace I need to go. Today, someone seemed to have organized the cosmos into a series of rooms. The rooms were connected by portals that opened and closed like the iris of an eye. It took a significant amount of breath and energy to get through a portal. Once I was through, it was a slower, more floating ride, giving me time to recognize and meet different tribes of ancestors. I often see dead people in these trance states and today was a red-letter day for the dearly departed. Some were deceased extended family members from this lifetime. Some were winged beings. Other rooms were filled with ancestors from ancient cultures. Each tribe imparted a different flavor of love and support. It felt like half the universe had showed up to say, "Hello, we love you. We remember you, even though you might not remember us. We all understand what you're doing and we're all here for you."

I laughed, I cried, I gasped in awe. But the ride I was on was not only happening inside my head—it was happening all through my body as well. Nan was standing beside the fMRI machine. She had asked me to squeeze her hand when I felt the beginning of an orgasm. I had first squeezed it when I blasted through the first portal. The more I breathed and set my intention to keep going further, the more the orgasm rolled through my body and the more frequently and intensely I squeezed Nan's hand. Nan was using her other hand to communicate to Dr. Barry the intensity of my orgasm. The more I squeezed her hand, the more fingers she held up. Nan told me she ran out of fingers less than halfway through my journey. I was in such an altered state I don't remember stopping. Next door, Dr. Barry and the fMRI technician collected their data.

The results were not available for some weeks. And yes, they revealed what I hoped and believed they would reveal. What I had experienced in that fMRI machine was indeed an orgasm. The insula, the hypothalamus, and the amygdala—regions of the brain typically activated during genitally induced orgasm—had all been activated. What I had been experiencing for the past 20 years had indeed been orgasms.

Depending on your perspective, my story of the fMRI scan could be a horror story, a kinky erotic scene, or a mystical experience. I experienced it as ecstasy. How did this extraordinary challenge turn into a transformational adventure? How, under all these incredibly unsexy and often terrifying conditions, was I able to have a scientifically verified orgasm that also qualified as a true ecstatic experience?

Looking back at the entire fMRI experience I was able to deconstruct it and examine the elements that led to the ecstatic conclusion.

I got through that frightening time by following my erotic intuition—the very intuition I'd been shaping, honing, and polishing for over 20 years. Over those years, I had learned how to trust my body and my spirit when pursuing the ecstatic. Without the ability to surrender to my intuition at each successive step in the process, I would never have found and sustained the courage to get through the scan, much less reach orgasm.

I also surrendered to my *need* for ecstatic experiences. Ecstatic experiences are necessary for my well-being. They are not happy accidents. I look for the opportunity to fly into the ecstatic part of any available experience. In this process, it took a constant and conscious recommitment to surrender—by this time it was surrender to the mystical process itself—to keep me flying through the ecstasy and to keep the ecstasy flying through me.

Surrender is not something one leaps into effortlessly or blindly. Surrender takes preparation. In the case of my fMRI experiment, it took months of soul-searching, planning, negotiating, setting boundaries, and building up my courage. Many people think this kind of preparation decreases spontaneity and therefore diminishes pleasure and ecstasy. I beg to differ. In my experience it's all the conscious preparation that makes possible true spontaneity and expanded ecstatic experience.

I was thrilled when I finally saw the edited documentary. It seems other people were, too. When the show aired on The Learning Channel I received hundreds of e-mails from people from all walks of life who wanted to know how they, too, could have breath and energy orgasms. I also received a few from people who'd been having breath and energy orgasms for years and were thrilled to finally have a name for the experience. Many of those who wrote to me had run into some form of roadblock on their erotic journey. Some had spinal cord injuries, gunshot wounds, clitorectomies, erectile dysfunction, or other physical conditions that prevented them from having genital orgasms. Others were experiencing loss of desire, boredom, incompatibility with a partner, post-traumatic stress disorder, celibacy by choice, and celibacy by circumstance. Whatever the cause or form of erotic roadblock, everyone asked if this new discovery that orgasms could happen without genital sex meant that there was hope for them. Yes, I answered, there is. There is hope for more than just an enhanced physical experience of sex. There is also new hope for expanded ecstatic experiences of everything our sexual expression gives us, such as freedom, intimacy, connection, release of tension, physical well-being, and spiritual connection.

So that's what this book is about—sex, but also much more than sex. It's about the infinite possibilities of ecstatic expression with which sex can provide us. It's also about how we can create ecstatic experiences when sex is not possible, available, or appropriate. Take a big, full, deep breath. Let's get started.

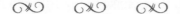

INTRODUCTION

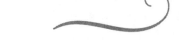

Permission and Possibilities

Imagine yourself at age 13 in science class. It's the first day of the school year. You've been eagerly awaiting this term because this is the year science gets really good. You're going to dissect frogs, learn about black holes, and create fascinating experiments in the lab. But on the first day, your science teacher walks in and says, "You are too young to learn about real science. All you need to know is that the earth revolves around the sun and gravity keeps you fastened to the earth. When you're older and married and working you'll find out all you need to know. Until then, don't do it. You could hurt yourself. And besides, God doesn't want you to know about science. He created everything and that's all He needs you to know. If you want to talk about science, talk to your parents. They are the ones who should be teaching you this stuff anyway."

How would you feel? If you're anything like me—or anything like most 13-year-olds—the first thing you'd do would be to run to the Internet and look up everything you could find about this forbidden thing called science. You'd search the TV listings for science programs and sneak books about science out of the library. Science would suddenly be all you thought about, all you talked to your friends about. What were the adults hiding? What didn't they want you to know? Science is a pretty involved subject, so as you pieced it together from questionable Internet sites and from the bits and pieces of information your friends had gathered, you'd get a lot of it wrong.

The last people you would go to in your quest for scientific information would be your parents. You'd remember how they had behaved when you'd first asked them about science several years ago. They'd given you vague, unsatisfying answers, and seemed embarrassed—as though they didn't know much about science either.

As you grew older you'd consistently grieve your lack of knowledge about science. You might occasionally still search for more information, or, you might have given up, deciding that you weren't really that interested anyway and you'd just muddle through with the little you did know.

What you may never realize is that the injustice done to you at age 13 was not the withholding of knowledge about science. The real unfairness was that the school did not teach you how to *learn* about science. There are very specific ways to approach science in order to discover its truths and vast possibilities. No matter how long we go to school, we do not learn all there is to know about any subject, including English, sociology, math, languages, and a myriad of others. But we do learn *how* to learn more about them. This is the real value of education: training minds how to learn more and how to grow with the new knowledge. If your education is lacking or was cut off too early, you may become educationally disabled in one or more subjects. Not only will you not know what you don't know—you also won't know how to learn it.

This has been—obviously—a long metaphor for the nature of sex education in most of the Western world. We don't know what we don't know and we don't know how to learn it. We take bad or incomplete advice because we are so eager for any information that can help us. This was certainly true for me. I learned absolutely nothing about sex from my parents or in school. Like most of us, I was completely self-taught. I made a lot of mistakes. At many points along the way, I became discouraged. I despaired of ever figuring it out or getting it right. It was not until I wanted to help others during the AIDS crisis that I realized that before I could change anything, I had to learn how to learn about sex. In the course of that part of my sex education, I learned the single most important lesson of my erotic life:

Each one of us is in the process of our own, unique, individual, sexual evolution.

There are an infinite number of erotic and ecstatic possibilities available to us at all points on our journey. The permutations and combinations of these possibilities create even more possibilities. It's vast—unimaginable, really. In order to realize our erotic possibilities we need to be able to choose which ones are right for us at each stage of our evolution. That's where the learning how to learn comes in. We need to learn how to *choose*—how to separate what's appropriate for us from all the things that aren't. And we need a way of figuring that out that is gentler and more effective than trial and error.

The people who were moved to write to me after my breath and energy orgasm experiment aired on The Learning Channel were motivated by two incentives: the permission to try something new and the Something More Factor. I discovered the Something More Factor when I first began teaching my breath and energy orgasm workshops. I'd ask people, "What are your orgasms like now and what would make them better?" The vast majority of people answered the second part of that question with some variation of: "I know there's *Something More* out there. I want to be able to let go and find it."

The Something More Factor is what drives us all in erotic—and spiritual—exploration. The longing for Something More impels some people to dive into the deep end of the pool of sexual excess, and stops others from even dipping their toes into the water. The search for Something More requires permission—from oneself or from some higher authority. Even if your family, society, spiritual community, or school encourages you to find Something More, you still need to be able and willing to give *yourself* permission to go find it. If and when permission is not forthcoming (or if it is expressly withheld) from higher authority, it is even harder to find within.

In 1989, author Louise Hay delivered a talk called the Totality of Possibilities. In it, she gave us permission—and encouraged us to give ourselves permission—to release old beliefs and fears. In doing so, she said, we would see that the limited set of possibilities we thought was available to us was a fantasy. In reality, we have an infinite number of possibilities to choose from—the Totality of Possibilities. Accepting this Totality of Possibilities is a key step on the way to finding our Something More. However, the concept of the Totality of Possibilities can be as frightening as it is liberating, especially when it comes to sex and relationships. The Totality of Possibilities includes a number of sexual activities that you may have absolutely no interest in and would never want to engage in. It includes types of people and styles of relationships (some of which you may have already experienced) from which you might run screaming. How do you sort through the Totality of Possibilities of sex and relationships to find the ones that are right for you? How can you explore sex and relationships without getting yourself into a whole lot of situations you would hate? It's that fear of the unknown—specifically the unwanted unknown—that can keep us stuck in the same old rut, doing the same old thing, and getting increasingly bored and dissatisfied.

That's what this book is about. It's about how to discover, nurture, expand, and embrace the authentic, ever-evolving, sensual, sexual you. It will teach you how to approach sex and relationships in a way that works for you no matter where you are in your sexual evolution. You'll get tools for solving the inevitable challenges that arise. You'll even receive permission to *not* do sex at all, along with guidance in how to find your ecstatic expression in other areas of life, if that's what's right for you. And you'll stop beating yourself up if your authentic sexual self doesn't match whatever limited set of expectations were imposed on you by your family, friends, partner, or the media.

As you might have guessed, this is not a traditional sex how-to book. It is not filled with sex tips and techniques and positions. There are many excellent books, blogs, podcasts, DVDs, and apps available today that provide accurate and inspiring information for more creative sex. If you already own some of these, there is no need to get rid of them; this book is not meant to replace them. Instead, this book will help you get the most out of them. Please think of this as a why-to book, a where-to-start book, a how-to-give-yourself-permission-to book, and a what-the-possibilities-might-be book.

The crucial first step to finding Something More is permission—permission to look beyond what you have now for something new and exciting, yet authentically you. In all my work, I help people bring their sex lives into alignment with the rest of their lives—their hopes and dreams and fondest desires. I help people reduce shame and become sex positive. I do that by giving people permission. I'd like to give you permission—and help you give yourself permission—right now with the following Sexual Permission Slip.

I originally wrote this permission slip as a performance for a high school sex education class. The students liked it so much they turned it into a call and response game. You can play a similar game at home.

Read each of the following permissions out loud. Repeat each one until you feel that you have successfully given and received permission from yourself to be, do, or have each item on the list. When you believe that you really have that permission, check off the box next to that item.

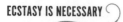

My Sexual Permission Slip

☑ I give myself permission to talk about sex.

❏ I give myself permission to talk about sex with the intention of learning something new, both about the person I'm talking to and about sex in general.

❏ I give myself permission to talk about sex as a safe, sane, and consensual act that brings health and pleasure to the world.

❏ I give myself permission to talk about sex as though it's really important—as important as politics and elections and human rights and stopping global warming and ending poverty and curing cancer. Sex is that important.

❏ I give myself permission to ask questions, dig deep, and find the meaning of sex—for me.

❏ I give myself permission to laugh. Sex is funny and sexual energy running through my body will often produce giggles—for no reason—for no reason other than that it feels good.

❏ I give myself permission to separate sex—temporarily— from all the things it's been glued to, like love, romance, and relationships. When I figure out what sex is—for me—then I can put it back together with things like love, romance, and relationships in combinations that are right for me.

❑   I give myself permission to do sex differently than my friends do, and to want different things from sex than my friends want.

❑   I give myself permission to keep sex just for myself.

❑   I give myself permission to not have sex at all.

❑   I give myself permission to figure out what my needs are before I have sex, when I am having sex, and after I have had sex—and to get those needs met.

❑   I give myself permission to take a risk—not a health risk, but an emotional risk, and even sometimes a physical risk. I give myself permission to let my soul get naked before my body does.

❑   I give myself permission to trust my instincts—even when (and perhaps especially when) other people don't like it.

❑   I give myself permission to say no and not explain why. I give myself permission to say yes and not explain why.

❑   I give myself permission to talk about sex. (Yes, that's right. Repeat it once more.)

CHAPTER 1

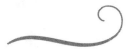

What Is Ecstasy?

Ecstasy is a universal human experience. It is not limited to those who are sufficiently spiritual, excessively sexual, or brilliantly artistic. Ecstasy happens to everyone, sooner or later, in one way or another.

But what exactly is an ecstatic experience? I have explored, written about, and discussed the ecstatic experience at great lengths, and I still have no easy explanation—no simple string of words that definitively capture its true essence. This is partially because the English language does not have an overabundance of words for intangible transcendent states. It's also because no two people experience ecstasy in exactly the same way. Since I am going to spend an entire book discussing how to create ecstatic experiences on a regular basis, we really ought to begin by figuring out how to talk about them. In order to find the right language, we need to ask the right questions. Questions such as: What is ecstasy? How do you know you've found it? What does it feel like? How can you get there and stay there?

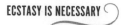
Having heard myself talk about this subject at some length, I wanted to know how other people experienced ecstasy. I formed an informal focus group of my Facebook friends and Twitter followers and began to take several highly unscientific polls.

The first question I asked was: What does an ecstatic experience feel like in your body/mind/soul? As you read these answers, make a note of any you've experienced.

For some people the ecstatic experience was expansive and active: It feels like . . .

- . . . my body has been engulfed by a pillar of fire.

- . . . God and Goddess are making love with each other inside of my body.

- . . . liquid sunshine is exploding out of me, touching everything and everyone around me.

For others, ecstasy was peaceful and grounded in the now:

- I feel warm, calm, at peace.

- I'm just there—nowhere else. My body is full of Life, and at the same time relaxed. My heart sings, and there is a huge YES!

One person described an ecstatic mind vs. an ecstatic body:

- An ecstatic experience in mind is bright, undisturbed, full of potential, lit, mysterious, known, wise. An ecstatic experience in body is still, grounded, strong, fluid, full, light.

For many people, ecstasy had a paradoxical quality, with two or more apparently opposite things happening at once:

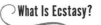

- It's the feeling of being everywhere and nowhere—being inside and a part of everything, and also floating far above it all.

- It's a feeling of going inside and going way out at the same time.

- Sometimes ecstasy feels like I am like a small strand of seaweed moving with the water. I feel myself moving toward the pulse of the water as well as moving a little away. Moving toward, moving away . . .

- Like nothing, and everything. Like smooth calm water during a rock concert.

The lack of boundaries was another common theme:

- There is absolutely no disconnection from my own energy and the energy of the universe and/or people around me. Boundaries are gone. It's all love, connection, pure. It's the true reality of oneness—which can sound cliché, but it is so very possible and alive in those moments.

- I feel beyond my physical body. I just feel pure energy. Pure consciousness.

- I feel like I'm floating in a borderless universe where only love exists. All fear is gone.

- Timeless, orgasmic electricity.

As was a feeling of heightened perception:

- I experience complete clarity and precision of awareness. With every heartbeat I can feel the blood move around my body. Every breath feels like a flood of energy.

- I am hyper-aware of sensations against my skin, sounds, smells, tastes, everything.

Many people felt a freedom to go beyond the ego-identified self:

- I experience complete and utter freedom. I feel weightless and take flight.

- I feel elation, rejuvenation, ease of breath, scintillating visions of aliveness.

- Sometimes I feel a buzzing; sometimes I lose time; sometimes I lose my sense of self; sometimes I lose my sense of solidity; sometimes I feel a quivering stillness. Sometimes it feels like an explosion of sensations; sometimes I feel raw and very real; sometimes a heightened lightness.

This often leads to a feeling of being a part of All That Is:

- It's like I'm making love to the particles in the air; like I'm warm honey pouring through bright, empty, boundless space.

- I am rooted to the world, and at the same time, connected to everything else. I am safe in the moment. It feels like I have always been and always will be.

- I feel an acceleration, a lightness of being, a swelling of consciousness and feeling of connection with Spirit.

- I fall into the "gap"—the space between all else.

One person summed it all up with:

- Ecstatic experience is the reason for human life on this physical plane.

It is interesting to note that no one described ecstatic experiences with words like *pleasant, pleasure, happy, nice*. Ecstasy is not a "feel good" or a "just good fun" experience. Ecstatic experiences disassemble us in some significant way and swirl our pieces back together again in new configurations. They give us a fresh perspective on who we are and what our place is within the greater universe. An ecstatic experience can shatter the glass ceiling of our limited possibilities, revealing a new unexplored galaxy. Paradoxically, not only will such an experience expand our Totality of Possibilities—but expanding our Totality of Possibilities will also increase our capacity for more ecstatic experiences.

Please glance through the descriptions of ecstatic experiences again. Which can you relate to, either in whole or in part? At what age did you experience similar feeling(s)? What were you doing at the time? If you have trouble remembering a specific feeling or incident, use your imagination. Can you imagine having any of these ecstatic feelings? When, and from what kind of experience?

The first experience in which many people recognize ecstasy is, unsurprisingly, sex and orgasm. Sex and orgasm are definitely among the easiest and most reliable paths to ecstasy, but they are far from the only paths. It's interesting to note that the people who answered the question "What does an ecstatic experience feel like in your body/mind/soul?" did not use sexual terminology or describe sexual scenarios. Although sex and orgasm can be the most popular routes to ecstasy, the ecstatic experience itself is not specifically sexual. I took a second, equally unscientific poll in my social media focus group. This time I asked, *"Please name ecstatic experiences other than orgasm and sex."* I was astounded by the response. Over 200 people submitted hundreds of answers in just a few hours. Here is a sampling of the results.

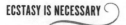

Art, Music

- Artgasms.

- Singing; jamming along with an amazing song; being sung to; toning; harmonizing.

- Playing music together with really good musicians. Watching and becoming one with a musician who falls into raptures of ecstasy while playing his instrument.

- I just reached a new level of artistic skill in rendering my work in ink. I got so high I spent 24 hours straight doing nothing but illustrations.

- Telling a joke on stage and feeling it land perfectly with the audience.

- Any sort of performance, such as public speaking or acting. I notice a sort of subtle energy-sex happening between me and the audience, or between me and the speaker if I'm in the audience.

- Being "didged" by live didgeridoo players.

- The sensuous, poetic words of Rumi, whispered to me in electrifying tenderness by my lover.

- To write, and just feel the words are true.

- Bon Jovi concerts—talk about transcendental experiences!

Birth

- Giving birth. Witnessing birth.

- Holding my first child for the first time.

- Holding my two little grandbabies for the first time.

Breathing

- Breathing into an ecstatic state.

- Breathing in the fragrance of a rose.

Connection

- Being with someone on some astral molecular level while on different continents.

- Real deep connection with a dear friend.

- Being alive, awake, and feeling the connection to all that is.

- Sitting quietly in the woods, around a fire, under the full moon, with a man with whom I connect on a deep spiritual level.

- To be met in the heart of my beloved—beyond words and concepts.

- To be seen as I am, and allowed to be just like that.

Dance, Drumming

- A dancegasm in a 5Rhythms/Wave workshop.

- Dancing all alone and naked in a pitch black room.

- Trance dancing. Club dancing. Dancing till dawn.

- Swing dancing with a great partner.

- Improvisational dancing. Belly dancing. Sexy Latin dancing.

- Dancing into the moment when the music starts dancing you and you're just riding the wave.

- Drumming to accompany a singer, dancer, or instrumentalist—especially around a fire.

Death or near death

- Being there when someone's spirit leaves their body.

- Seeing my wife open her eyes after days on life support.

Drugs

- Especially hallucinogens.

- Flying through the "portal" to meet my ancestors and guides on a DMT trip.

- Sipping a good martini or Manhattan and enjoying the glow.

Falling/being in love

- That electric look you get from someone who is in love with you.

- Marrying the man of my dreams and still being deeply in love years later.

- Making up after a fight.

- Making a special someone happy.

- Rare, precious, bygone moments shared with another, when just for a moment I believed I could and would

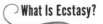

live truly magically with that person, in spite of time and places.

- Getting a puppy for the first time.

Food

- Chocolate, chocolate mousse.

- Italian food eaten in Italy.

- Food soaked in butter.

- The first bite of perfectly seared foie gras.

- The sweetness of strawberries contrasted with the bitterness of dark chocolate.

- Eating a perfectly ripe, fresh pear.

- Tasting a perfect Roquefort cheese together with a sweet white Bordeaux wine.

- Poached eggs on toast.

- Eating mackerel-flavored ice cream at MoVida in Melbourne, Australia.

Laughing

- Laughing until I cry.

- Laughing my ass off.

- Gigglegasms.

- Playing with small children and letting them climb all over you, laughing and giggling!

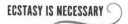

Nature

- Watching shooting stars above Sedona or over the inky, dark Pacific on a moonless night.

- Sunset on a beach, when the sky goes rosy and the ocean a deeper blue.

- Feeling the cold sparks of fresh snow falling on my body as I relax in a warm, wild hot spring.

- Sitting on the beach with my yoni open to the water, greeting one another.

- Breathing air after a long climb up a mountain.

- Dancing along the rim of a volcano.

- Meeting a manatee.

- Floating naked in the fluorescent night ocean, with the moonlight dancing on my body, surrendering to her soft, wet, caressing undulations. Surrendering, trusting, ecstatic . . . ahhhhh home!

- Running naked in the forest on a warm, full-moon night.

- Swimming with the dolphins and making eye contact with them.

Political action

- Pumping out rhythms in an anarcho-samba street band (our refrain, Drop Bush Not Bombs!) in the middle of Third Avenue. Hundreds of thousands of us occupy the streets. It's February 15th, 2003, and New York City is refusing to cooperate with Bush's plans to invade Iraq.

- Participating in a hot political debate on live TV.

Religious/spiritual practices

- Prayer.

- Meditation in all its forms, including but not limited to: Zen, active, still, drumming, gonging, and toning.

- Every breath I take—if I am really aware.

- A great Kundalini yoga workout.

- Merging with angels or source.

- Singing gospel music in church.

- Praise dancing.

- Sufi spinning.

- Coming out of a five-hour sweat lodge.

- Reading tarot cards and feeling the flow as the spread unfolds and every card is exactly perfect.

Sports

- Swimming, snorkeling, scuba diving.

- Riding a boogie board on rolling turquoise waves.

- Bungee jumping, skydiving.

- Being "in the zone."

- Sailing.

- Breaking a board in self-defense class and feeling the energy flow through me.

- Hula-hooping.

- Running.

- Being a child sitting on the swing and going high, high, higher!

Touch

- Certain kisses and hugs that stop time.

- Massage by a very strong man/very strong woman.

- Channeling Reiki and seeing "Reiki bubbles" floating around the room—with my eyes open.

- A long deep kiss that takes me to a place I have never been.

- Large piles of people all being gently and joyously tactile.

- Barely there kisses.

- Being at one with a massage client.

- Lomi Lomi or Kahuna massage.

Traveling

- Without an itinerary.

- Walking the streets of NYC any time of the day and night.

- My first plane ride as a child.

And more!

- A steamy hot shower after a long day at the computer.

- Finding a bargain on a cool antique.

- Finding an awesome shoe sale.

- Taking a risk and having it pay off.

- Hallucinations! Delusions! Death! Roller coasters! Being five years old! That scene in the movie where the villain gets it, bang! Finally beating your big brother at something! Being swept up in the madness of the crowd! Ending sentences with exclamation points!

- Watching fireworks.

- A really, really, really good cry.

In addition to the routes to ecstasy listed above, some people reported finding their bliss via routes less traveled. For thousands of years people have practiced rituals and ceremonies—many of them as part of initiations or devotional practices—that involve pain, supplication, ordeals, and bloodshed. In the past 30-odd years many of these practices from the past and from indigenous cultures have been reinterpreted and reinvented by modern ecstatic explorers. Some of these adventurers responded to this question as well. Here are some of their paths to ecstasy. (Remember, the totality of erotic and ecstatic possibilities may include activities in which you have absolutely no interest. If you think you would find reading about rituals involving pain and blood disturbing, give yourself permission to skip over the items on the last half of this list.)

- Riding the Cyclone at Coney Island. (The Cyclone is the legendary roller coaster that has been delighting and terrifying riders since 1927.)

- Being seen naked, especially for the first time by someone, or by large numbers of people.

13

- Fire walking. (Fire walking is the act of walking barefoot over a bed of hot embers or stones.)

- Fire spinning. (Also known as fire dancing, fire spinning is a performance art that involves the manipulation of objects on fire. Typically these objects have one or more bundles of wicking, which are soaked in fuel and ignited. Spinners and dancers use hoops, fans, balls, sticks, whips, and poi—a pair of arm-length chains with handles attached to one end, and bundle of wicking material on the other—as flaming performance props.)

- Getting pierced or tattooed.

- Pain.

- Truthful, connective deep BDSM play. (BDSM stands for Bondage/Discipline, Dominance/Submission, Sadomasochism.)

- Ball dancing. (Weights—including fruit, balls, bells, or other decorations—are hung from temporary piercings sewn on to the upper back, chest, and arms. The weights pull and tug as the dancer dances, releasing powerful endorphins.)

- Participating in a hook pull. (A hook pull or energy pull is a ritual based upon the Native American Sundance Ritual, in which participants are pierced in the upper chest with two sharp hooks. Ropes are tied to the hooks and then to a stationary object such as a tree, or to the hooks of another participant. By gradually increasing the tension on the piercings as one pulls, one shifts one's energy toward an altered state.)

- Being single tailed and caned. (A single tail is a bullwhip or signal whip with a single braided thong. A cane is a flexible woody stalk, similar to bamboo. Both can be enjoyed by people who like to receive stingy sensations.)

- Participating in a hook suspension. (A hook suspension is a ritual in which the participant is hung—or partially hung—from hooks pierced through the flesh in various places around the body.)

Ecstasy is available through so many avenues! I point this out to clients when they claim that joy, pleasure, or ecstasy is not possible in their lives because, for some reason, sex is not available to them. Yes, orgasm and sex are hugely important, and for many people sex and orgasm are either the easiest or the only ways they know to access an ecstatic experience. But ecstatic experiences are available in a myriad of other ways. When you increase your ability to create ecstasy out of the stuff of ordinary life, all of your ecstatic sexual experiences grow deeper. And when you learn how to create ecstatic experiences with orgasm and sex, you can also learn to create ecstasy from the substance of the rest of your life.

Some people who read the lists above will ask, "Are these really ecstatic experiences? Aren't they just rushes of adrenaline?" Certainly there is a difference between a purely adrenaline experience and an ecstatic experience. As a culture we do consume a great deal of what I call faux ecstasy. The buzz we get from working too intensely, drinking too much caffeine, and multitasking are just three examples of ecstasy substitutes that many of us consume on an all-too-regular basis. People get similar highs from food, drugs, alcohol, shopping, drama and gossip, extreme sports, violent entertainment, fast cars, thrill rides at amusement parks, and Internet pornography. However, it's a mistake to think that an adrenalized state can never lead to an ecstatic one.

Often, an adrenalized state precedes an expanded transcendental state, such as the nervous frenzy someone might work themselves into when they are about to try a new sexual activity, or have sex with a new partner. In situations like these, adrenaline

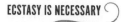

is part of the chemistry that helps such a person transform their fear into excitement and eager anticipation. Similarly, for most people, riding the Cyclone roller coaster simply produces an extreme adrenaline high. But if conditions are right, and the rider has the skill, that ride—or the afterglow from the ride—can become an ecstatic meditation.

Which brings us to the question: How do you know you are really having a "true" ecstatic experience? My friend Robyn had an experience that dramatically illustrates the difference.

> Some months ago I fell into trance while dancing to drums. I felt beyond my physical body. I felt like pure energy, pure consciousness. That sensation lasted some minutes. Suddenly, I felt an inexplicable fear and I fell down. The feeling of fear caused me to try and control the experience, and when I did, I stepped right back into all my limitations, all my conditioning. The secret to ecstatic experience is to really allow myself to go into the movement and flow of pure energy.

You may be thinking, "Well, all this talk of ecstasy is nice, but I am nowhere near an ecstatic experience. I just want more satisfying sex and a better orgasm. How is all this talk of ecstasy going to help me?" Whether your needs and desires seem modest or extraordinary, the path of ecstatic and erotic evolution is the same. You are where you are now, and you desire Something More. Ecstasy is a relative experience, and it's available in steps. It is not a fixed destination in some faraway land, reachable only after you lose weight, clear all your chakras, learn the entire Kama Sutra, spend years in therapy, meditate extensively, study with a guru, and find a better partner.

Ecstasy is not a goal. Ecstatic experiences may be found everywhere along countless paths to self-love and personal growth. This means that the only thing you have to change right now is any lingering belief that ecstasy can't happen to you.

Ecstasy is not "better" than sex. It is not more spiritual, more evolved, or more acceptable than "just sex."

I despise the phrase "just sex"—as in, "It's not love; it's just sex." Or, "It's not a relationship; it's just sex." Or, "What's the big deal? It's just sex." The dismissal of sex as some lower form of energy or lesser activity is a denial of both our physical reality and our spiritual potential.

Sex is an expression of who we are. It's not simply a description of physical qualities—as in "She's so sexy!"—or quantities—as in "Boy, I sure am getting a lot of sex lately." It's not even an activity—as in, "I'm going to fuck your brains out." Sex is energy—our life-force energy—and it is expressed in every area of our lives. There is no difference between going-to-work energy, eating-dinner energy, taking-out-the-trash energy, and sexual energy. It's all life-force energy. Because the same life-force energy that flows through us also flows through every living thing on the planet, we are in an ongoing erotic relationship with all of life all the time. How much of it we see, feel, or appreciate is dependent upon how much of this energy we have learned to recognize, accept, and allow.

Everything we experience during the years we live on planet Earth is interpreted through our bodies. The emotions we feel, the thoughts we think, and the physical sensations we have are all accessible to our consciousness only because we have bodies. Our bodies and brains are programmed to gravitate toward things that feel good and to avoid things that feel bad. Whether it's an item of clothing, a new car, a piece of music, or a romantic relationship, we are constantly making choices based upon whether something turns us on or turns us off. We are, by design, erotically based beings.

If we choose to, we can eroticize anything and everything. If you don't believe me, check out the *Encyclopedia of Unusual Sex Practices*, which describes over 750 items or practices that turn some people on. Our natural ability and inclination to eroticize explains why some people can have an orgasm by kissing their partner's high-heeled shoe, why others can become intensely turned on when they are tied down, or how I was able to have an energy orgasm in an fMRI machine.

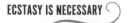

One of the easiest ways to understand and explore this broader definition of sex is to expand our definition of orgasm. Orgasm could simply be defined as a sexual climax attained by stimulation of the genitals and other erogenous zones. But as we've seen—and science has now proved—orgasm is not an experience limited to the genitals. It happens in the brain as well.

Orgasm also has a releasing and relaxing effect on the entire body, and it regularly produces altered states of consciousness. Therefore, orgasm could be more broadly and accurately defined as a release of tension and an expansion of energy flowing through the body/mind and connecting us to spirit. Science is reluctantly beginning to acknowledge the truth of the hypothesis for which orgasm researcher Wilhelm Reich was imprisoned in the mid-20th century—that ecstasy in the form of total orgasm is *medically necessary* to the health and well-being of the human body.

If the experience of orgasm is not limited to our genitals—and if we can even orgasm without genital stimulation—what other kinds of alternative and expanded orgasms are possible? You have probably experienced several of them even if you did not recognize them as orgasms at the time. For example, remember the last time you had one of those unstoppable laugh attacks that started with one funny incident or joke and ballooned into a gigglegasm? You were gasping for breath, your diaphragm was spasming, and you wondered for a split second if it was possible to die from laughing too hard. How did you feel at the end of that gigglegasm?

Or how about the last time you let all your rage just fly? The more anger you released, the more there was to release. You screamed and swore and pounded and yelled so loudly that your throat was sore afterward. Remember how you felt after that angergasm? And how about tears? Have you ever cried so long and so deeply that you felt like you were crying for every sad thing that had ever happened anywhere on the planet? Do you remember how you felt after that crygasm? Was it similar to how you felt after an angergasm or gigglegasm?

Emotiongasms are total experiences. You allow your body to express emotions without trying to suppress or change them.

18

Allowing an emotion to become orgasmic releases the hold it has on us. The story behind the emotion is dissolved. During a gigglegasm we may forget what initially made us laugh. We simply become the laughter. In a crygasm we go beyond the initial impetus for our tears and simply become the crying. And in angergasms we scream out the original source of our rage and just become pure power expressing itself. We emerge from these experiences cleansed, open, empty, and reborn.

What's more, expanded orgasmic experiences are not limited to a handful of emotiongasms. Look at all the ways people were able to reach ecstasy in the Facebook and Twitter poll earlier in this chapter. There were dancegasms, hula-hoopinggasms, massagegasms, kissgasms, yogagasms, chocolategasms, and lovegasms, just to name a few.

Our bodies are hardwired for ecstasy. Whether or not your definition of sex involves your genitals; whether or not you are in a relationship—romantic or otherwise, monogamous or non-monogamous; whether you are able-bodied or differently abled; you are a sexual being pulsing with erotic energy. How you choose to experience your eroticism and find your unique form of ecstatic expression is completely up to you.

I invite you to think of making love the way Wendy-O Matik defines it in her book, *Redefining Our Relationships*:

> Making Love = Being Loving: anything and everything that you put your heart into, including intercourse, a hand shake, kissing, a love letter, a peace offering, S/M, art, music, masturbation, fetishes, fantasies, a phone call, a warm embrace, whatever pleases you, whatever feels good, the sky is the limit. I dare you to count the ways you can single–handedly make love to the planet or yourself or your best friend or your new lover.

I invite you to think of it all as love. I invite you to think of it all as sex.

For clarity's sake, from this point forward in the book when I use the word sex I'll be referring to any conscious expression, experience, or act of sex, eroticism, and/or ecstasy.

Think of yourself as an ecstatic, erotic explorer. All that means is that you want Something More and have made a commitment to find it. You need no extraordinary qualities or talents. I asked people who were experienced in both sexual and spiritual exploration—people who were not only explorers themselves, but also well-versed in helping others find their ecstasy—to tell me the qualities shared by ecstatic, erotic explorers. Here are their answers. How many of these qualities do you already have? Which can you imagine cultivating?

- Compassionate

- Courageous

- Creative

- Curious

- Desiring, hungry

- Enthusiastic

- Flexible, resilient, open-minded

- Honest

- Loving

- Mindful, present, conscious

- Passionate

- Persistent, determined, committed

- Playful, innocent

- Respecting, self-respecting

- Self-loving

- Humorous, funny

- Sensual

- Willing to listen, to communicate

And there's more. My colleague Tessa Wills adds that it is important for all of us beginning or expanding our erotic exploration "to be able to sit in an easy relationship with our shame." Notice that she did not say that we had to eliminate all our shame before we could begin. We simply have to be willing to allow it to appear every now and then. At each step of the way we are likely to encounter either a little or a lot of shame. Shame must be accepted, forgiven, and gently moved beyond. If you wait to eliminate all your shame before you take the next step in your sexual evolution, you'll never take that next step.

In a similar vein, it's helpful to be willing to feel uncomfortable occasionally. The ecstatic path is ultimately rewarding, but moments along the way are likely to be awkward, exhausting, or confusing. A willingness to be vulnerable and look silly is absolutely critical. Above all, the ecstatic path requires a commitment to self-knowledge. You have to know yourself in order to be successful as an erotic explorer. The good news is that one gets to know oneself increasingly well as one walks the path.

In the pages to come I'll show you how to create the conditions that allow more and more of your experiences and encounters to be opportunities for and invitations to ecstasy. We will start with self-knowledge. In the next chapter you'll have the opportunity to discover—or to re-examine—your values, your needs, and your desires with the intention of finding out exactly who you are and where you are—today—in your own personal erotic evolution.

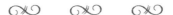

CHAPTER 2

In Search of Your
Authentic Sexual Self

Let's pretend you've just bought the car of your dreams. It's sleek and shiny and exactly the right color. The genuine leather seats and polished dashboard exude the ultimate new-car fragrance. You pull out of the dealer's lot and happily drive away. When you get home, you open the glove compartment, eager to find the owner's manual and learn all about your precious new vehicle. To your dismay, the manual does not say "Mercedes SLK300." It says "Generic Automobile Manual." It points out that you have tires, doors, windows, and mirrors. It's filled with crazy-making advice such as, "If the flashing symbol on the dashboard looks something like this, it could either mean that you are out of gas, or that your tires need inflating, or that your engine is about to seize."

You'd be pretty upset, right? You'd spend the next few weeks and months tentatively trying to get to know your car by trial and error. Just when you thought you'd gotten it all figured out, some new mysterious flashing light would throw you into a panic as you tried to evaluate what it meant and if it were serious. If you had owned several different cars of various makes before this one, you would have a better idea of how cars work and a better idea of what the warning signals might mean. If this were your first car, you'd most likely be mystified and maybe even terrified.

This is pretty much how all of us navigate through sex and relationships. Very few of us are trained mechanics. Almost all of us have learned by trial and error. The information available to us, especially when we are just starting out, is dangerously one-size-fits-all.

In this chapter you'll begin to understand how you're built as an erotic, ecstatic being, and how you run. In subsequent chapters you'll discover exactly how you are wired for sex and relationships and what your personal warning signs look like. You'll learn how you operate and what reference manuals and tools you might need for optimum care. On top of all that, you'll finally be able to communicate this information effectively to others so that they can love and enjoy you more easily and more passionately.

So get a blank notebook and we'll get started. If you like, you can title it: *My Ecstatic Sex and Relationship Operating Manual: Instructions, Troubleshooting Tips, and Advice on Lifetime Maintenance.* Give your notebook a title that invites you to write in it and read it. As you work through the simple exercises in this and in the following chapters, you'll begin to discover who you authentically are as a sexual being and what you most want and need from your relationships right now. And *right now* is the key phrase. We are all in a lifelong process of sexual evolution. It begins the day we are born and lasts until the day we die. As in any evolution, we shift and change constantly. Sometimes your progress may seem slow or even nonexistent. At other times changes will happen overnight. At 40 years old we may have desires for things we never even knew existed when we were 16. At 50 we may wonder if we will ever feel sexual again. At 60 we may be more sexually active than we were in our 20s. The process is all very personal and individual.

This is where your sex- and relationship-operating guide comes in. As you create your operating guide, your authentic sexual self will reveal itself to you. What do I mean by your authentic sexual self? I mean the you that has been shaped and motivated by your values, your needs, and your desires. When you know who you are and what you value, need, and desire, it's a snap to select the most exquisite choices from the menu of infinite erotic possibilities. You'll save yourself time, anxiety, and heartache and you'll experience a great deal more joy, pleasure, love, and ecstasy.

Before you can start to imagine, appreciate, and choose from your totality of erotic possibilities, you'll need to know three things about yourself:

1. What do I value?

2. What do I need?

3. What do I desire?

The answers to these three questions will set you free. Instead of swimming in an ocean of guilt, doubt, and trial and error, you'll have reference points for each of the choices and decisions you'll face on your path of erotic expansion and transformation.

Let's start with a short series of warm-up questions. Don't think too hard. Write down the first thing that comes to mind.

Why do you do sex?

What does it give you? What's the delight?
What's the big payoff?

Were you able to easily articulate an answer for each of these? Or did these questions seem odd? Or difficult? Was your first thought, "Well, everybody knows that, right? We all do sex for the same reasons."

The truth is we don't all do sex for the same reasons. In another of my highly unscientific polls, I asked several dozen people from different walks of life these same three questions. Here are some of their answers:

- To connect/communicate with another person.

- To connect with myself.

- To connect with my animal nature.

- To get out of my head and into my body.

- To scratch an itch—the need to come.

- To turn my brain off.

- To release tension.

- To lighten up.

- To find out what is happening inside of me.

- To look better—sex is especially good for my skin.

- To escape, to avoid, to procrastinate—especially when I'm overwhelmed.

- To bring myself into the present moment.

- To give the other person pleasure.

- To feel wanted and needed.

- To explore different sides of my personality.

- To give completely and to surrender completely to someone else's giving.

- For the adventure.

- For mystical experiences/mystical connection.

- To experience altered states.

- It's a natural painkiller. It stops the pain of my fibromyalgia.

- It's a legal high/non-addictive high.

- It's one of the only ways I enjoy being present in my body.

- To make a spiritual connection with another person and take both of us from this real world into a different dimension.

- It's the glue that binds my marriage together.

- To open my heart.

- I like the noises.

- It makes me feel grounded.

- I like being told I'm beautiful and worthwhile.

- To forget how much life hurts.

- It's the most authentic time I have with myself.

- For intimacy and touch.

- And yes, one person answered, "I am trying to have a baby."

So, why is it useful or important to know what you and your partner(s) love about sex? Here's a personal example. I do sex for the mystical experiences—for the connection to all the disembodied beings and spirit guides I meet in erotic trance. I love altered states of consciousness, and nothing has ever beat sex and orgasm for consistently delightful—and often profound—travels through the cosmos. I have a partner who values sex as passionately as I do—for a completely different reason: she gets high on the intense intimate connection with her partner. With such different reasons for doing sex, we had our challenges in finding a way of creating sex together where she felt the connection she needed and I did not feel constrained. But as we grew to know more exactly what our differences were, it was easier to find creative solutions to this apparent incompatibility. For example, we spent more time connecting in the earlier stages of sex, so that when I went blasting off into the stratosphere at orgasm my partner did not feel so abandoned. She knew I'd be back and we could reconnect again soon. She even learned how to jump on my magic carpet and ride with me occasionally, and I've learned more about honoring our togetherness. When we bring greater awareness to our deepest longings, it becomes easier to find ways to accommodate seemingly disparate reasons for enjoying sex.

The longer I talked to people about the true value sex had in their lives, the more I could see a through line. The majority of people reported that they liked sex because of some form of connection. What differed was what they preferred to be in connection *with*. Some people wanted to be in connection with another person. Others wanted connection with God/Goddess/All That Is. Some wanted connection with an aspect of themselves, while others wanted a feeling of purpose, or aliveness, or love, or inner peace.

I personally subscribe to the theory that all human desire for connection is a desire for connection with the divine—for connection with God/Goddess/Universe/All That Is. Sex and sexual energy allow us a direct physical experience of the divine within ourselves and with others—a direct connection to the center of everything. As humans, one of our strongest connections to this source energy—one of the few ways we can touch it, feel it, and smell it—is when it is embodied in another human during sex.

Humans do sex for hundreds if not thousands of other less lofty reasons, including many of which are situation-related:

- I wanted to celebrate a birthday or anniversary or special occasion.

- I was curious about what the person was like in bed.

- I wanted to be popular.

- I wanted to say "thank you."

- I was horny.

- I wanted attention.

- My partner kept insisting.

- I wanted to keep my partner from straying.

- The person made me feel sexy.

- I got "carried away."

- I wanted to make up after a fight.

- The person was too hot to resist.

- I hadn't had sex for a while.

- The person had beautiful eyes.

- I was drunk.

- And so many more . . .

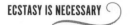

But these are not the fundamental reasons we desire sex. Each time we have sex, we are hoping to fulfill the deep longing for that most essential personal reason that we need/love/want/crave sex—which you have begun to discover, simply by answering a few warm-up questions.

So, now that you know why it is that you do sex, let's move on to three questions that will help reveal your authentic sexual self.

What Are Your Values?

Have you ever had a disagreement with a beloved that was different from any other argument you've ever had? No matter how hard you tried, you could not understand their point of view on "The Issue" and no matter how hard they tried they could not understand yours? It may have sounded like your beloved was speaking some obscure dialect of a dead language. The words sounded familiar, but they made no sense at all. And no matter how carefully you phrased your feelings, they made no sense to your beloved. They appeared to be listening, but they certainly weren't hearing you. This kind of sudden-onset, painful misunderstanding, once started, often gets repeated every time you try and talk about "The Issue." If this has happened to you, then you and your partner are most likely experiencing a conflict in values.

Your values are essential to who you are. They are the core organizing principles you use to live your life. Your values are like the operating system on a computer, constantly running in the background of whatever application you might be working in. They influence every choice you make and every interaction you participate in. They are a cornerstone of who you are.

Values are defined in various ways by different people. An academic, an entrepreneur, and a therapist, for example, are likely to have three different ideas about what values are, how to arrive at them, and how to apply them. There are also many different kinds of values: personal, business, social, legal, educational, organizational, spiritual, vocational, physical, financial, family, religious . . .

just to name a few. Some people say that people, places, and things cannot be values—values can only be higher feelings, ideas, and beliefs such as freedom, joy, and love. Others say that anything that really matters to you—anything you use as a guiding principle to focus your life—can be a value.

The more deeply you examine your values, the more you link all areas of your life to your *highest* values. Your life becomes more meaningful and fulfilling. In order to be happy at work, for example, your personal values must align in some way with the organization's business values. In order to be happy in a relationship, your personal values must align (or be able to be aligned) with someone else's values. You may have examined your values in the past. You may re-examine them on a regular basis. Right now I am going to invite you to examine your values for the purpose of discovering yourself in sex and relationships.

In this context, we'll understand "values" to mean: 1) the people, places, or things that mean a great deal to you; and 2) the underlying principles, feelings, or beliefs that those people, places, or things represent.

For example, several people may list money as an important value in their lives. Upon closer inspection, one person may value money because it provides them with the freedom to travel around the world, another because it provides for their family's needs—and yet another because they love to give it away to causes they believe in. Money, in these cases, fulfills three different core values: freedom, family, and generosity. It is likely that many of the people, places, or things that each of these three people value also satisfy these three core values.

In the following exercise you'll discover your core values. Core values form the bedrock that supports your life. You may be able to list dozens of people, places, and things that you value, but your core values are probably no more than six.

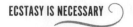
EXERCISE: FINDING YOUR VALUES

First we'll discover what matters to you. Then, we'll discover the core values represented by the things that matter to you.

Step One: Open your notebook/journal to a blank page. Answer the following question: Who or what is really important to me?

Don't think too hard. Release the impulse to give answers you think you *should* give.

It may help to look at your life as though you were an outside observer. How do you spend your time, your money, your energy? In what areas of your life are you the most disciplined and organized? What's in your home, on your walls, on your shelves? What do you think and talk about? What are your goals?

Write down 6–10 answers.

(If you find this challenging or difficult to do on your own, do the exercise with a friend, lover, or anyone with whom you feel a comfortable, safe connection. Your friend will keep asking "Who, where, or what else is really important to you?" until you have come up with 6–10 answers.)

Now, rank the 6–10 items in order of importance with the most important as number 1. For example, let's say you came up with these 6 answers:

- Car

- Career

- Trust

- Partner

- Respect

- Love

Which of these is most important to you? Which is the second most important? If this is difficult, your friend can help you by following this script for each of your answers. Place a check next to each answer in the list you've made in your journal.

What is more important to you? Car or Career?
What is more important to you? Car or Trust?
What is more important to you? Car or Partner?
What is more important to you? Car or Respect?
What is more important to you? Car or Love?

What is more important to you? Career or Trust?
What is more important to you? Career or Partner?
What is more important to you? Career or Respect?
What is more important to you? Career or Love?

What is more important to you? Trust or Partner?
What is more important to you? Trust or Respect?
What is more important to you? Trust or Love?

What is more important to you? Partner or Respect?
What is more important to you? Partner or Love?

What is more important to you? Respect or Love?

Then count all the check marks to reveal your top six values in order of their priority or importance to you. If there are two values with the same number of checks, go through the same process to find the most important.

If you started with more than six values, eliminate all but the top six.

Now let's move on to Step Two, where you will discover your core values.

Step Two: Let's say that "My Partner" came out as one of your values. Ask yourself (or have your friend ask you):

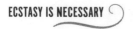

What does "Partner" mean to you? What does "Partner" give you?

Your answer: Closeness.

What does "Closeness" mean to you? What does "Closeness" give you?

Your answer: Love

What does "Love" mean to you? What does "Love" give you?

Your answer: Trust

What does "Trust" mean to you? What does "Trust" give you?

Your answer: Honesty

What does "Honesty" mean to you? What does "Honesty" give you?

Your answer: Certainty

What does "Certainty" mean to you? What does "Certainty" give you?

Your answer: Security

Let's assume that this is your final outcome. Meaning, when you ask "What does Security mean to you or give you?" the answer is "Security." This is your core value, which you are trying to get met through a partner.

Some values on your list, such as Trust, or Respect, may be not only a value, but also one of your core values. If, for example, when you are asked "What does Trust mean to you?" you answer "Trust," you have arrived at a core value.

Follow the same process for all six of your values. Use your intuition—when you get to what seems to be the end of a line of inquiry, let it be the end. You'll know when you have reached your core value.

More than one of your six initial values may lead to the same core value. For example, both "Car" and "Career" might lead to a core value of Freedom, or Prosperity.

Step Three: How closely are you living your life according to your core values? Take a moment to reflect. Using a new page in your journal, on a scale of 1 (meaning I'm not living at all true to this value) to 10 (I am in complete alignment with this value) make note of how closely your life matches your values. This is not an exercise about judging or criticizing yourself. None of us will always be completely in alignment with all our core values. Rather, this is an exercise in awareness. Now, how might your core values apply in the realms of sex and relationships?

Here's an example: Let's say you have been in a relationship with your partner for the past five years and all is going well. One day they decide they want to travel the world for a couple of months alone. Your reaction: *This is a disaster! You absolutely must not go! I won't survive!* When you know your values, you know that it's not your partnership that is being threatened, but your core value of security.

Or, let's say you are short of money. You and your partner each have a car. You live in a city with decent public transportation and you rationalize that you could make do with one car between you. Yet, every time you think of selling your car to save on gas, repairs, and insurance, you feel angry, anxious, or sad. What is upsetting you is not your sense of poverty. Your core value of freedom is being challenged.

Do you see how knowing your values can help you take better care of yourself? And how knowledge of your values can help you to understand why you (or someone you love) might react intensely when a seemingly minor event occurs? When we know our core values we can more easily get to the root of the problem and seek out solutions that realign us with the actual value

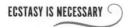

being threatened. We can also comfort ourselves by giving ourselves what we really need instead of what we think we want.

OPTIONAL EXERCISE: ANOTHER METHOD FOR FINDING YOUR VALUES

Below is a list of common personal values. Although I think the previous exercise is a more accurate way of discovering your core values than picking them from a list, I offer them as an inspiration and an example of all the many things we value.

On your first pass through this partial list it's likely you'll see many values that feel important to you. Please be selective. Try to pick no more than 20–25. From that, reduce the number to ten. Finally, choose your six most important values.

Abundance	Bliss	Community
Accomplishment, achievement, success	Bravery	Compassion
	Broadmindedness	Competence
Accuracy	Calm, quietude, peace	Competition
Acknowledgment	Challenge	Concern for others
Adaptability	Change and variety	Connection to God/ Goddess/ Universe/All That Is
Adventure	Chastity	
Affection	Cheerfulness	Continuous improvement
Artistic expression	Children—inspiring/ encouraging/educating them	
Authenticity		Cooperation
Balance and harmony	Cleanliness, orderliness	Courage
		Courtesy
Beauty	Close relationships	Creativity
Being responsible and dependable	Collaboration	Curiosity
	Comfort	Decisiveness
Being the best	Commitment	Delight
Belonging	Communication	Dependability

Dignity

Discipline

Discovery

Discretion

Diversity

Duty

Dynamism

Eagerness

Ecological awareness/ responsibility

Economic security

Ecstasy

Effectiveness

Efficiency

Elegance

Endurance

Energy, vitality

Entertainment

Enthusiasm

Ethical practice

Excellence

Excitement

Extravagance

Fabulousness

Fairness

Faith

Faithfulness

Fame

Family

Feeling part of some-

thing bigger than myself/nature/God

Fierceness

Financial security/in- dependence

Fitness

Flair

Flexibility

Freedom

Friendliness

Friendship(s)

Frugality

Fun

Gallantry

Generosity

Global view

Goodwill

Grace

Gratitude

Gregariousness

Happiness

Hard work

Harmony

Having a family

Health

Helping other people

Holiness

Honesty

Honor

Hospitality

Humility

Humor

Hygiene

Independence

Individuality

Influencing others

Ingenuity

Inner peace

Inner vision

Innovation

Inspiring others

Integrity

Intelligence

Intelligent thinking/ reasoning and analyzing

Intensity

Intimacy

Intuition

Involvement

Job tranquility

Joy

Justice

Kindness

Knowledge

Leadership

Learning

Liberty

Logic

Longevity

Love (romance)

Love (unconditional)

Loyalty

Making a difference

Maturity

Meaningful work

Meeting the needs of others

Merit

Meticulousness

Mindfulness

Modesty

Nature

Neatness

Nutrition

Obedience

Open-mindedness

Openness

Optimism

Order (tranquility, stability, conformity)

Organization

Originality

Outrageousness

Passion

Patriotism

Peace, non-violence

Perfection

Personal development/growth

Personal responsibility

Philanthropy and charity

Playfulness

Pleasure

Popularity

Power

Practicality

Privacy

Professionalism

Progress

Prosperity

Public service

Punctuality

Purity

Quality of work

Quality relationships

Reason

Recognition

Relaxation

Reliability

Religiousness

Reputation

Resourcefulness

Respect

Responsibility

Responsiveness

Romance

Sacrifice

Safety

Satisfying others

Security

Self-control

Self-direction: doing what I love, choosing my own goals

Self-reliance

Self-respect

Sense of purpose

Sensitivity

Sensuality

Service

Serving a higher purpose

Sexuality

Sharing

Simplicity

Skill

Solving problems

Sophistication

Speed

Spirituality

Stability

Status

Strength

Success, achievement

Surprise	Tranquility	Vision
Surrender	Transparency	Vitality
Teamwork	Trust	Warmth
Thoroughness	Truth	Wealth
Thoughtfulness	Understanding	Winning
Thrift	Uniqueness	Wisdom
Tidiness	Unity	Wittiness
Timeliness	Usefulness	Wonder
Tolerance	Variety	
Tradition	Virtue	

What Are Your Needs?

Some would say that the only true human needs are biological: We only *need* to breathe, drink, eat, sleep, urinate, and defecate—everything else is some form of desire. Although that may be technically true, it's not very helpful. We all have intense desires that we experience as needs. I know that I have very real needs that go beyond basic survival. And I know that getting these needs met has a higher priority than getting my wants and desires satisfied.

When our desires are not met we may be disappointed, frustrated, and/or angry. When our needs are not met we can become physically, emotionally, or mentally incapacitated.

All humans share a similar set of needs—much as we share our DNA—yet the details of each person's need-set are unique. Your needs may have been shaped by an incident that happened in your childhood, or by something as recent as a breach of trust in your last relationship. Just as sometimes you don't recognize one of your core values until you realize you're not living in alignment with that value, sometimes you don't know what your basic needs are until they are not met.

For example, my friend Leigh succinctly explained why she

was breaking up with her boyfriend, "I need a boyfriend who re-members my birthday," she declared. Obviously, the fact that he forgot her birthday was not the only reason she was breaking up with him, but this simple declaration expressed a basic need that she had realized was not being met: the need to feel special, to be known and seen, especially by someone she loved.

In the field of psychology much has been written on the sub-ject of human needs. One of the most popular and most refer-enced scales of human needs was developed by Abraham Maslow, a professor of psychology at Brandeis University and a founder of humanistic psychology. Maslow said that once basic physical survival needs were met, humans had a hierarchy of other basic needs. Maslow's Hierarchy of Needs states that we must satisfy each need in turn, starting with the first, which deals with the most obvious needs for survival itself. Once the lowest level of needs has been met, we can move on to the next level—safety and security—and so on up the pyramid. If the things that satisfy our lower levels of needs are swept away, we will no longer be con-cerned with our higher-level needs. For example, if an earthquake destroys your home, disrupts the distribution of food, and shat-ters the pipes that carry water through your town, you will not be concerned about your reputation at work.

Maslow's basic needs are:

- *Biological needs:* these include oxygen, food, water, sleep, and a relatively constant body temperature. They are the strongest needs and must be met first.

- *Safety and security:* this includes personal security, finan-cial security, health and well-being, and some sort of safety net in case of accidents, illness, or unemployment.

- *Love and belonging:* these include social groups, profes-sional associations, family relationships, friendships, intimate partnerships, extended families, sense of tribe, and close confidants.

- *Respect and esteem:* the need to be accepted and valued by others. According to Maslow, there are two types of these needs: the need for status, attention, recognition, and respect from others; and the need for confidence, competence, independence, and self-respect.

- *Self-actualization:* When all four of the preceding sets of needs are met, the need for self-actualization is activated. Maslow described self-actualization as a person's need to be and do that which the person was "born to do." It's the desire to become more and more what one is, to become everything that one is capable of becoming.

Beyond these five levels of basic needs, Maslow described higher levels of human needs, such as needs for understanding, aesthetic appreciation, and spirituality.

Where does sex fit into all of this? Sex is often considered a biologically imperative need; however, unlike food, water, and oxygen, humans can survive without sexual activity—the human race cannot—but individual human beings can and do. Over the course of human history, our expectations and needs for sex have changed. As illustrated by the long list of answers to my "why sex" question, sex has not been a purely procreative act for a long time. Sex has evolved into one of the ways we get many of our basic needs met—including safety and security, love and belonging, respect and esteem, and self-actualization.

Not all human needs concerning sex include the presence of other people. We have erotic needs that can be fulfilled outside of our relationships with partners and lovers. Yet as humans, we all have needs for relationships with others and most of us prefer to get our sexual needs met in a relationship. Our relational needs influence how we contact and connect with other people. Simply put, my relational needs are what I need and want from you when I am in relationship with you.

In their book, *Beyond Empathy: A Therapy of Contact-in-Relationship*, Richard G. Erskine, Janet Moursund, and Rebecca

Trautmann define seven categories of relational needs: security, validation, acceptance, mutuality, self-definition, making an impact, and expressing love.

I have expanded this list of needs into an exercise to help you figure out your most important needs in relationships with others. Many of our most urgent relational needs are the same across all our relationships. But, it is likely you also have needs that are specific to certain relationships. For example, your most important needs in relationship with your mother are likely to be different from your needs in relationship with your lover. Often you don't notice that you have a need until that need is not being met. For example you may not realize how important your need to be heard is to you until you find yourself in a relationship with someone who can't seem to remember what you told them yesterday.

So let's begin the process of recognizing our unique needs, both in life and in relationship to others. The following is based upon a list compiled by my colleague, sex and relationship educator, Corey Alexander, and expanded upon with contributions by my Facebook and Twitter focus groups. Using a new page in your journal, go through this list and make note of the needs that seem the most urgent to you, then rank them in order of importance. You may need to do this several times for different areas of your life and for different relationships, e.g., work, lovers, friends. For example, you may have one set of needs for friends in general, and another somewhat different set of needs for each specific friend. If a specific need applies to a specific relationship, make note of that as well.

Also, feel free to add words to each item to make the need specific to you. For example, to "To be seen in my complexity . . ." you might add ". . . especially with regard to my passion for both opera and punk rock." Or "To feel listened to and heard when I talk to _____ about my reluctance to join them in _____." In doing this you will discover not only your basic needs but how they are playing out in specific relationships.

Be selective. Resist any temptation to pick all—or the majority—of needs on the list. Choose only your most important, most urgent needs. You may find that you have several urgent needs in one category, but few or no needs in others.

Lastly, know that your needs will change over your lifetime, sometimes in a relatively short period of time. Don't spend too much time trying to unearth all your oldest, deepest, unmet needs. Identifying your "needs of now" will be more useful.

1. Security. In Maslow's hierarchy, the needs for survival and safety must be met before a person can respond to any other kind of need. This is usually true in relationships as well. We need to feel that we won't be attacked, swallowed up, or abandoned. We need to feel safe and free from threats of shame and humiliation. It's important to know that we can be who we really are in relationship and show all of ourselves without fear of losing the respect and affection of the other person or persons.

Common needs relating to security:

- To feel safe.

- To feel cared for.

- To be free from emotional and/or physical pain.

- To know where I stand.

- To feel connected to other(s).

- To have a support system for times of trouble and joy.

- To have time together.

- To have needed information, to be kept in the loop, to hear it first, to get a heads-up.

- To feel at ease, peaceful.

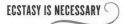

2. Valuing. This is the need to be understood, valued, cared about, and thought worthy. It includes unconditional positive acceptance of our feelings, fantasies, needs, and identity by another person. When this need is met we have a sense of being normal and acceptable just as we are.

Common needs relating to valuing:

- To be treated with respect.

- To be seen in my complexity.

- To feel valuable, valued, appreciated.

- To feel desired, wanted. To be the object of another's desire.

- To receive physical affection.

- To be listened to and heard.

- To feel that my feelings are accepted unconditionally.

- To be able to succeed, make mistakes, be vulnerable, be strong.

- To be thought trustworthy.

3. Acceptance (by a stable and protective other person). In this need, not only is acceptance itself important, but so are the qualities of the accepting person. This is the need for acceptance by a strong, stable, reliable, consistent, and dependable person. We want to feel that we have a protective trustworthy person in our lives who looks out for us.

Common needs relating to acceptance:

- To trust in another's word, commitment, integrity, and adherence to agreements.

- To know that someone will be patient with me if I mess up.

- To be able to rely on someone's authenticity and sincerity.

- To know that I can rely on someone for emotional support, and to be able to ask for help if I need it.

- To know that I will be given the benefit of the doubt.

- For someone to be totally present with me.

- For someone to have spiritual awareness and compassion.

- To feel someone is loyal to me.

- To be able to hold someone accountable for their actions/ promises/responsibilities.

4. Mutuality. This is the need to be with someone who understands what you are experiencing because they have experienced something similar, in real life or in imagination. This is the need not to have to explain everything fully, to be understood without having all the right words, and to find someone who shares and supports our view of the world.

Common needs relating to mutuality:

- To be understood.

- To have emotional outlets, emotional intimacy.

- To enjoy mutual support of goals.

- To share a vision for the relationship.

- To have language to describe the relationship and define who we are to each other.

- To share daily life with someone.

- For all members in a family/network to be intimately connected in some consensual manner.

- To communicate effectively.

- To share playfulness, laughter, fun, and joy.

5. Self-definition. This is the need to experience and express our own uniqueness and to have the other person acknowledge and respect that uniqueness. It's the mirror image of the need for mutuality, i.e., the need to be different as contrasted with the need to be similar. Self-definition is our need to be a separate being with individual preferences, interests, and ideas.

Common needs relating to self-definition:

- To preserve my identity and be my authentic self.

- To have my own work (paid or not) outside the relationship.

- To have privacy, confidentiality.

- To have my own space, solitude, free time.

- To adhere to my own ethical system.

- To dream a future/have goals/be passionate about something.

- To be able to change, grow, shift, mutate, and otherwise evolve.

- To define (and redefine as necessary) who we are to each other in relationship.

- For all members in a family/network to have mutually acknowledged clear boundaries.

6. Making an impact. Impact means having an influence on another in some desired way. It's the need to attract the other's interest and attention, to help them see something differently or do something in a new way. Being able to influence others helps us feel useful and important to others. We want to see the effects of our impact and know that something has happened in response to our input.

Common needs relating to making an impact:

- To feel useful.

- To help others change and grow.

- To feel that I matter to others.

- To be able to give support in bad times and good.

- To feel like I make a difference.

- To create safety and comfort for others.

- To provide healing for others.

- To care for others.

- To motivate others.

7. Expressing love. This is the need to give love. It may be expressed as gratitude, showing affection, or doing something nice for another person. It's important that these expressions of esteem and appreciation are accepted and welcomed, even if they are not perfectly chosen or perfectly timed. In short, it's the intention that matters most.

Common needs relating to expressing love:

- To have sex, play, pleasure, touch, skin time.

- To touch, hug, give and receive physical affection.

- To give kindness, care.

- To give unconditional love.

- To be passionate.

- To be creative and spontaneous.

- To have control or surrender control.

- To provide emotional outlets/emotional intimacy for another.

Reading through this list can be overwhelming. If that's what's happening for you, put the book down, go do something else, and come back to this list as many times as you need to make your unique list of relational needs. Then, ask yourself:

Am I getting these needs met?

If not, who, where, and what might be able to meet these needs?

Am I willing to compromise getting any of my needs met, and if so, which ones and just how far?

Do I see a relationship between the needs I just named and the values I discovered in the previous exercise?

These are questions you can use again and again. Consider them tools for relationship maintenance. Here's how two of my clients used them.

Faye saw an immediate connection between one of her core values—beauty—and her need for sex, pleasure, and touch. Faye had been seeing Phil for eight years. They tried living together for a year, but it wasn't right for either of them, so they went back to living apart and dating. They saw each other regularly, but had sex infrequently (every two or three months). And they never spent the night sleeping together. She lived in a lovely apartment, but Phil did not like her bed. He said it was too hard, so after cuddling with Faye until he thought she was asleep, he slept on the sofa. Faye tried staying at Phil's apartment, but his bed was small and lumpy and the apartment was cramped and run down, with mold and chipped paint on the walls. Faye tried everything from sexy lingerie to trips away to entice him into more regular lovemaking, but nothing worked.

After seeing her values and needs in writing, Faye realized that although the sex was very good when they did have it, and although she and Phil were compatible in all other areas of their lives, this relationship met neither her most important needs nor her core values. She decided to let the relationship transition into a friendship and began to look for a romantic and sexual relationship elsewhere.

Allowing your needs and your values to inform each other can help you solve all sorts of long-standing sex and relationship issues.

Doria was looking for a long-term relationship but couldn't see how to make one work. She became increasingly bored with her lovers after they had sex for the first time. At 38, she felt immature. Unsurprisingly, two of Doria's core values turned out to be freedom and variety. When she understood that her desire for sexual variety was actually an expression of her core values, she was able to figure out other ways to line up her sexuality with her values. Doria discovered she had a deep need to give love and pleasure to another. She decided that she could create sexual variety by finding endlessly creative ways to give pleasure to a single lover. She also decided that although she was looking for a long-term relationship, she did not want to live with anyone, thereby allowing herself the feeling of freedom she cherished.

Now let's add the last major piece to this process of self-discovery: your desires.

What Are Your Desires?

We create our lives—however badly or well—through the per-
petual process of desiring. A desire can be as modest as craving a
chocolate, or as grandiose as hungering for unlimited power and
wealth. Desire can be the spark that leads to a loving, fulfilling
relationship, or the harbinger of megalomaniacal lust.

The nature and purpose of human desire has been hotly debat-
ed for centuries. In many organized religions, desire is interpreted
to mean sexual desire and is either discouraged, condemned, or
restricted. In Buddhism, desire (sexual or otherwise) is believed to
be at the root of all human suffering. In fundamentalist American
Christianity, which descended from the Puritans, sexual desire is
seen at best as a distraction from productive work and at worst as
the destroyer of one's relationship with God.

Yet, we all desire all the time. Esther Hicks (conduit for the
non-physical intelligence she calls Abraham) is fond of saying that
new desires are being born within each of us every minute. When
a desire is young, its fulfillment can seem impossible. As we focus
on it and put effort into the creation of it, our desire may seem
distant, but it's no longer impossible. Every step we take brings us
closer to the fulfillment of that desire, until one day, that once-
distant, improbable desire is simply the next logical step. This is
why getting what we desire is not always as satisfying as the process of wanting it. The reward of desire fulfilled is not entirely in
the satisfaction of *getting* what you desire. Much of the satisfaction
is in the memory of what it took you to get you there.

Joan had always wanted to see the great pyramids of Egypt.
She found a bargain on exactly the tour she wanted to take, but
she was still short $2,000. Joan just *knew* she was supposed to take
this trip. She saved and prayed and repeated positive affirmations.
She told everyone she knew about the trip. Her excitement was
infectious. Her friends threw her a fund-raising party in a local
bar where she not only received several hundred dollars, but also
met the very attractive brother of a former college roommate. Still
short of the money she needed, Joan took a second, part-time job

for a child welfare agency. In that job she learned valuable skills in social media marketing, made two new close friends, and found a renewed sense of purpose. One of her new friends decided to replace her lightly worn luggage and gave Joan an entire set of nearly new bags for her trip. By the time Joan was standing in front of the pyramids in Egypt, she was not only amazed by the astounding sights in front of her, but also in awe and gratitude for all the love and miracles she had experienced along the way.

Joan's odyssey from initial desire to realization could have been obsessive, difficult, and alienating. But Joan held her desire lightly. When she wondered if she'd be able to raise the money she needed, she thought, "If for some reason I cannot raise the money in time for this particular trip, I know that an even better tour of the pyramids will come along at an even better price." She did not torment herself with her goal. She was committed to it, but not obsessive about it. Obsession is the enemy of creative desire. Obsession leads to tunnel vision—we can only see our goal and the single path we think will get us there. We become completely oblivious to the Totality of Possibilities of ways in which our desire could be fulfilled. This is equally true with regard to sexual desires.

Most of us have experienced some sort of obsessive desire, if only as a teenager. We see someone we are attracted to and become convinced that our desire for them is true love—that they are our one and only soul mate and without them our lives will be forever empty. We go to outrageous lengths to get them to notice us or to love us. We persuade friends to participate in elaborate plots to bring us together with our beloved. We ignore a dozen attractive and available lovers simply because they are not the one we are obsessing over. This kind of unhealthy desire may even lead to stalking, murder, and suicide.

The seven deadly sins—lust, gluttony, greed, sloth, wrath, envy, pride—are all examples of desires taken to extremes. The fear of falling down the "slippery slope" into an obsession with sex has kept many people with harmless erotic desires from trying to satisfy them. The ecstatic experiences we are yearning for are not obsessive compulsions—unless we approach those ecstatic

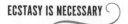

experiences unconsciously. Our yearnings for Something More range from harmless desires inviting us into greater aliveness, to the callings of our soul pulling us toward transformation.

It is just as dangerous to ignore our desires as it is to obsess about them. Whatever we repress will ultimately express, often causing far more damage than if we had just satisfied the desire in its early stages. Children subjected to severe discipline and control often grow into reckless, freedom-seeking missiles that wreak havoc on themselves and others. Adolescents who are punished and shamed for any expression of their sexuality may become sexually compulsive in one form or another. Those who don't act out, often turn their stress inward, causing emotional and physical illnesses.

Everyone has a unique relationship with their desires. Some embrace them wholeheartedly; some are fearful. Some perceive a significant difference between sexual desire and other forms of desiring. For others, they are one and the same. Again I polled my Facebook and Twitter focus group. I asked: *What is the nature of your desiring? Does a sexual desire have a different quality than other desires?*

Some people thought there was a significant difference. My friend Lin wrote:

> It's quicker, easier, and more socially acceptable to publicly satisfy a desire for other things—like chocolate! You can even do it in a conventional workplace. Sex, sexuality, and sensuality are all so mired in guilt and shame in this culture (especially when I was coming of age) that I learned early that sexual desire was a dangerous and unacceptable thing to acknowledge openly. It took a lot of work to combat that training and be able to claim myself as a sexual being—and be okay with that. However, unlike many of my other desires, I still prefer to keep that one less public.

Some agreed that there was a difference between sexual desires and other desires, but their reasons varied:

- Sexual desires can be fulfilled with nothing but a little sweat and imagination. Not necessarily so with other types of desires.

- I have a much harder time ignoring sexual desires than other desires and I'm 62 years old. Can you imagine what it was like when I was younger?

- Sexual desires can lead me to the ecstasy of the divine in degrees and ways that no other desires can.

- Sexual desires feel more physically powerful to me. An average, nonsexual desire feels like something to shoot for. "Hey, it'd be nice if I had lobster tonight, but I will be fine if I don't have it." Sexual desires carry an urge. I think my sexual desires do this because they connect to some emotional bits of me that have powerful needs.

- Only sexual desire makes me wet.

- I'm normally much clearer about other desires. My sexual desires seem to come at me sideways.

- Sexual desires are more fun.

Other people thought that all desires were essentially the same:

- To me, basic/primal desires like wanting that yummy chocolate cookie or striving to do well on a test strike a visceral chord within me to "go and get it . . . NOW!"

- I take all my desires as simply natural inclinations for some satisfaction. Having sex is on the same level as sharing a really good event with someone who enjoys it as much as you do—a meal, a party, or a day trip.

- Desire is a wish or wanting to enjoy something pleasurable in life no matter what it may be. Desire is the longing for connection—to commune with spirit, other people, and the planet. It is both a gift of gratitude and an inspiration for more to be grateful for!

Some people had positive relationship with their desires:

- Desire is what moves me to action in all areas of my life. I can't live fully without it!

- Desire is the emotional quality that gives me "that" feeling down the back of my neck just before the bonds are released and I begin to fly.

- Desire is as divine as its satisfaction.

Others had an uneasy relationship with their desires—at least at the moment:

- Desire is one of the main reasons society is living in pain and suffering. Most people desire what they cannot get, from money to fame to lust. Desire has no practical use but to create false, egotistical, wishful-thinking fantasies.

- It depends on when you ask me. Right now desire is vulnerability. It's a minefield, fraught with peril. Ask again tomorrow.

Whatever your unique relationship with desire, your desires are mutable. They will change and grow over the years more frequently and rapidly than your values and needs. It's not necessary to know all your desires. You just need to know how to hear them, feel them, and allow them.

What are some of your desires—erotic and otherwise? Have you ever been asked—in a romantic context or any other—"What would you like?" and not been able to think of a single thing? We cannot name our desires unless we have given our desires the opportunity to reveal themselves to us. Desires often show up most readily in our dreams, fantasies, and imaginations. Here is an exercise to help you get in touch with some of your desires.

EXERCISE: YOUR EROTIC MOVIE

Imagine yourself as the character in an erotic movie. You get to define "erotic" any way you like. Your movie can be sexually explicit, intensely romantic, or cast with beautiful, leather-clad creatures cracking whips. Please do not judge yourself for your choice.

Please get out your notebook and answer the following questions:

If I were the lead character in my erotic movie . . .

What would the view be from my bedroom?
What would I wear?
What would I eat?
If I could choose anyone, living or dead, who would my lovers be?
How would I like to be touched?
What three sexual activities would I excel at?
What three new sexual activities would I try?
Who would my friends be?
What would people say about me?
What three places would I go that I have never been?

Write down how this exercise made you feel. Was it easy for you? Fun? Challenging? Something else entirely? Wait a week and repeat the exercise. Compare your feelings and your answers.

It is in the realm of desire that the Totality of Possibilities of sex and relationship really begins to reveal itself, which can be frightening. Yet it is in the realm of our desires where we can find the first glimpses of our erotic transformation and ecstatic future.

In the following chapter you'll use your values, needs, and desires to form a firm but flexible foundation—and a safety net—from which you can launch into your next phase of erotic growth and ecstatic expansion.

CHAPTER 3

Safer Sex for
Ecstatic Explorers

Have you ever thought, *Why is it that sex seems easy, fun, plentiful, and pleasurable for everyone but me? Why does everyone else seem to have sex that is filled with physical pleasure, intimate connection, and a sense of wonder? What's wrong with me?*

If you have ever thought this—or are thinking it now—welcome to the majority of the adult and teenage population. Some of us live with this as a persistent question, but we all ask ourselves this at one time or another. Even someone in an open relationship with multiple, loving, sex partners can feel as though they just aren't as fulfilled as the couple next door seems to be. We live in a culture where commerce and the media have a vested financial interest in convincing us that everyone is having more and better sex than we are. If, they claim, we just buy their pill or product or service, we, too, can have the kind of ecstasy that "everyone else" is having.

Have you ever stopped to think, "Wait, if everyone else is having such great sex, why would these companies spend a fortune trying to reach a nonexistent market?" Well, of course, they wouldn't. Their product pitches are successful because there is an awful lot of sexual dissatisfaction out there.

For many people sex is, or has become, more of a problem than a pleasure. For some people sex is painful: physically, emotionally, or socially. Still more people have lost interest in sex—perhaps because they are bored with having the same kind of sex with the same person over a long period of time. And some people were simply never that interested in sex to begin with. They wonder, why is sex is such a big deal to everyone else? Many people feel broken, abnormal, crazy, or ostracized from the mainstream culture because they don't feel the way they believe everyone else feels about sex.

In truth, we are all looking for satisfaction of a longing that is far deeper than a better orgasm. We want to satisfy not just our body's longings, but also our soul's. We want ecstatic experiences—transcendent experiences—peak experiences.

Name and describe one or more ecstatic experiences you have had.

Imagine, name, and describe an ecstatic experience you'd like to have.

(Go back to Chapter 1: What is Ecstasy? if you need inspiration.)

Jack Morin, sex therapist and author of *The Erotic Mind* has done extensive research on peak sexual experiences. Morin says that a peak sexual experience is the result of just the right combination of safety and risk. I couldn't agree more.

My ecstatic experience inside the fMRI machine was a perfect example of walking that edge of safety and risk. Everything about that experiment—the medical scenario, the claustrophobic setting, the removal of my jewelry—was risky to the point of terrifying me. So before I actually attempted the breath and energy orgasm, I had numerous safety precautions in place. I had Sarah for emotional support. I had developed trust in the researchers and I had effective ways to communicate with them while I was inside the machine. I had familiarized myself with how the experiment would proceed. I had an escape strategy. And I had my blindfold and earplugs. Having examined my fears and then put conditions in place to soothe them, I was able to let go into the experience itself. Although I certainly was not able to eliminate all my fears, I was able to accept them as tolerable traveling companions on my journey.

The idea of exploring new sexual possibilities can bring up a lot of fear. Before we can enter into situations where new ecstatic possibilities might be created, we must first establish safety. This chapter will provide you with nuts and bolts advice on how to create the physical and emotional safety you'll need to move forward ecstatically.

Erotic safety is the not the sort of safety your mother wanted for you when she called after you, "Be careful!" as you left the house. If your mother was anything like mine, that "Be careful" meant "Don't do anything risky." Was there a parental figure in your life who told you not to take risks? Let's call that person "Mom." As you no doubt remember, the risky things your mom warned you about were always the most fun. In the realm of ecstatic erotic experience, they still are. Later in this book I'll be encouraging you to take risks—all the risks you'd like. And I promise you it will be fun. But first, I want to ensure that you know how to create safety for yourself—a kind of safety that is more like a solid foundation than a protective shell.

In the previous chapter we looked at our values, our needs, and our desires. Now let's take a moment to look at some common sexual fears so that we can create appropriate safety precautions that will allow us to take erotic risks.

Our sexual fears can silently pile up over the course of our lives until we find ourselves facing a wall standing between where we are now—and where we'd like to be. Our fears may be rooted in early personal experiences, including traumas such as abuse, incest, and rape. However, many far less traumatic experiences can lead to fears that we carry consciously and unconsciously into every new erotic encounter.

For example, were you ever ridiculed for your lack of sexual experience in an early sexual encounter? Maybe you were teased about some imagined physical shortcoming? You may have been traumatized by a string of inconsiderate lovers, or wounded by some post-lovemaking criticism about your performance. Perhaps you have been punished for being too sexual, or not sexual enough. Maybe you've been told that you are abnormal, sick, or perverted for expressing a harmless desire.

Sometimes we are aware of these sexual fears and traumas. Sometimes we don't know we have a fear until it leaps up and paralyzes us in the middle of an encounter.

Some triggers of fear in sexual situations have nonsexual roots. Here's a story that illustrates one of those.

I had set up for the final ritual of a weekend-long sex magic workshop. I am fond of didgeridoo music and was playing one of my favorite selections for this ritual. I had also lit a number of candles, as I intended fire to be the primary symbol for the raising of erotic energy. As I began the ritual, one participant left the room, followed by her husband. I was concerned, but her husband gave me a reassuring nod as he left with her, so I proceeded with the ritual. Within a couple of minutes, her husband reentered the room, gave me a second reassuring nod, and sat down. We finished our ritual. When it was over the husband went quietly back out the door and returned with his wife, Melanie. Melanie explained that as a teenager, she had had an extremely frightening experience in a ritual involving a Ouija board. The combination of the music, the candles, and the nature of this particular sex magic ritual had triggered some very scary feelings. Melanie knew she could not participate in this ritual but did not want to ruin the experience for others, so she left before her fear was out of control. She came back when she was calmer and things were once again safe enough for her.

One potent source of our fears is the warnings about sex we receive from our culture, subculture, our religious institutions, some medical professionals, and our family. Sex is profoundly unsafe in our society. Recently I read news reports of a local government using obscure and irrelevant zoning ordinances in an effort to prevent a sex education center from opening in their town. Sex is apparently so dangerous we even stop ourselves from talking about it intelligently with the intention of increasing our knowledge. Every day someone is victimized by ignorance or prejudice. Men who derive erotic and emotional satisfaction from dressing as women can be socially ostracized—even beaten or killed if they are discovered in public. Teenagers are thrown out of their homes for being gay or transgender. As I write this, the Ugandan parliament—urged on by a group of American radical evangelicals—is seriously considering a bill to execute gay people. For a brief period in the 1960s and 1970s, things were different. Sexual experimentation and freedom were actually valued by a large percentage of society. But this did not last long. Sex went from good to bad again in the 1980s when a conservative government, in collaboration with the popular media, used the fear of AIDS to whip society into a fresh new hysteria about sex.

In a culture where people's sex lives are used against them like atomic weaponry, stepping out of line can cost you dearly. Having sex in an unusual way, or having sex with too many people or with the "wrong" people may result in serious—even violent—social repercussions. It can cost you your relationships with your partner, your children, your family, or your employer. The erotic and sexual values of love, compassion, tenderness, respect, and freedom are sadly out of step with society's values of strength, work, profit, and conformity.

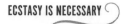

When it comes to sex, does your religion, community, or society show any interest in your values, your needs, your desires, or your ethics? Or is it more interested in your morals? Running a society on morality is a highly subjective endeavor. Who is to decide what is moral, i.e., what is right and what is wrong? You? Your neighbors? Government? God? The person who shouts the loudest?

Take a moment to think or write about the ways in which your sex life has or has not been accepted by your family, your neighbors, your community, or your culture.

Judgments about sexual behavior can traumatize a person for life. We inherit many of our fears from preceding generations who suffered social punishment by stepping out of line sexually. It was not until my mother was dying that I found out how horribly scarred she had been from a love affair gone wrong. My mother—who had been the most rabidly anti-sex person I knew and from whom I hid everything about my sexual life for my entire life—had in fact been a very sexual young woman. She had carried on an extremely passionate sex-and-love affair with a man who went away to war. When he returned after the war, he dumped her. She had expected marriage. In 1940s small-town America, this meant that she was damaged goods. I can't even imagine the shame and pain she went through.

On top of it all, I was never able to ask my mom about that, because she was not the one who told me this story—my father did. In the course of telling me that story, my father told me repeatedly how he did the *right* thing by denying her repeated requests for sex until they were married. He had clearly been holding these judgments throughout their 57-year marriage.

As adolescents, we may castigate our parents for their prudery, or laugh at their warnings about inappropriate sex, but we often unconsciously craft our own sex lives in the erotic model we saw when we were growing up. If we do radically—or even slightly—depart from that model, we may feel guilt and shame, and attract partners who reinforce that guilt and shame. Of course there are exceptions.

During the sexual revolution of the 1960s and '70s, an entire generation threw off the sexual constraints of preceding generations. For us to achieve that level of sexual freedom today, we must first make a conscious commitment to cultivate our authentic sensuality and sexuality. Without that commitment, we will tend not to venture much beyond the erotic backyard of our parents and immediate family. Without conscious commitment to our Something More, fear will cause us to retreat back into familiar territory. We may not be completely fulfilled, but we feel safe.

EXERCISE: MESSAGES ABOUT SEX

Open to a blank page in your notebook and answer the following questions:

What was the loudest message you heard about sex when you were growing up? That message could be from anyone or anything—your family, your school, your church, your community, or the media.

In what ways does this message influence your life? How has it affected the choices you've made about sex and relationships from adolescence till now?

Growing up, I received two equally strong, diametrically opposed messages. From my mother I heard a very direct message: sex will ruin your life. The message was delivered in many variations, but the bottom line was always that sex is dangerous. Having sex—or even looking sexy—would ruin my reputation, prevent success in my career, and even destroy my chances for future happiness.

The other equally potent but more indirect message I received was from television and movies. That message was: Sex will get you everything you'll ever want—money, glamour, a fabulous career, and gorgeous lovers. Sex was very confusing for me as a teenager and young adult. I was an extremely sexual young woman, but every one of my sexual encounters was fraught with conflict. To this day I still have moments when I wonder whether a new sexual encounter will provide the answer to all my spiritual questions, or simply be more trouble than it's worth.

Those were my conflicting messages about sex. You may discover that some big, bad message you received about sex is at the root of a particularly strong fear or turnoff. Here's a story that illustrates the lingering effect of such messages.

I asked a college audience to think about the two questions in the exercise above. My lecture was sponsored by a campus peer-counseling, sex information group. In our meeting before the lecture, the members of the group expressed their excitement not only about the lecture, but also about the breath and energy orgasm workshop that would follow. I explained that I would teach them how to use breath and a visualization to gradually take themselves into an orgasmic state. Everyone would remain fully clothed and no one would be touching themself or anyone else.

When we got to the workshop room after the lecture, I was surprised that one of the most enthusiastic members of the peer-counseling group was not present. I asked if she was okay and one of her friends assured me she was, and that she would see us later. When I finally met up with her she apologized for not attending the workshop. She explained that during the lecture she realized that her loudest message about sex had been that she must never, ever be sexual in public. Having just unearthed this old message, she felt uncomfortable about practicing breath and energy orgasms in a room with 75 of her classmates. She was very clear that this was a limitation she wanted to move beyond, so she'd spent the two hours we were all in the workshop journaling her way out of this belief.

It's helpful to look at the assumptions that we have made about sex. These assumptions function like urban myths—we've acted as if these assumptions were natural laws for so long that it never occurs to us to wonder if they are actually true. Three myths that pop up again and again in my workshops and in my sex coaching practice are:

1. Sex = Love;

2. Sex = Relationship;

3. Orgasm = Genitals.

You may have your own unique assumptions, but we'll use these three as an exercise in assumption busting. Let's take the last one first—Orgasm = Genitals—because it's the easiest one to debunk. As we've seen, genital orgasms are just one kind of orgasm in a vast universe of orgasmic possibilities. Even science agrees with us. Let's move on to two more big assumptions that may not be as easily debunked, but debunk them, we shall.

Sex = Love. No! No! No! Sex is sex and love is love. We don't need to be in love in order to have sex. We certainly don't have sex with everyone for whom we feel love. For many people, sex and love is *sexandlove*—an inseparable package. Any suggestion of sex without soul-mate-level romantic love, or outside the love of a committed relationship or marriage feels threatening or wrong. Other people feel relieved when they can separate sex from love, especially from romantic love. They feel a sense of freedom in the possibilities inherent in a more expanded notion of love and loving relationships.

Any connection between sex and love is a wonderful thing, especially when romance is new and feelings of love and sexual enthusiasm ricochet off and intensify each other. The question is: What is the nature of the connection between sex and love—for *you*? What relationship between sex and love makes you feel

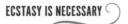

safe and valued? The question is not, for example, whether monogamous relationships are better than non-monogamous relationships—or vice versa—but whether or not you have made your choice consciously, and that your choice is in line with your values and your needs. Pondering these notions will help deconstruct any Sex = Love assumptions you might be living with.

How about Sex = Relationship? It's a myth. So—one day we will find the one person/soul mate whom we love, and we will make a commitment to be sexually faithful to them for as long as the relationship lasts. Really? Is there only one person for you out there? Really? What if that was just one of a thousand options? What if you could love multiple partners in a vast variety of different relationship styles? What if having regular sex with your primary partner was just one option? What if you could even have loving, committed romantic relationships without sex? What else might be possible? Giving some quality thought to these questions will help you let go of any Sex = Relationship assumptions that might be limiting you.

The ability and willingness to question all assumptions and limitations is crucial in making your ecstatic experiences safe and possible. While it is not advisable to smash through legitimate boundaries (which we'll discuss in depth in the next chapter), it is appropriate to ask, "Is this true for me? What would I need to make myself feel safe if I wanted to explore beyond this myth, assumption, or limitation?"

Busting a myth or shattering an assumption does not mean walking away from your values, your needs, or your desires. Rather, it's about taking a manageable risk for the purpose of consciously creating an authentic erotic reality for yourself.

The Resilient Edge of Resistance

Jack Morin notes that if we feel too safe, too comfortable—if there is no risk at all—there is also likely to be no turn-on at all. For a peak experience—or even just a hot time—there needs to be some element of risk. Anxiety can and often does function as an aphrodisiac, providing it is not so intense as to be paralyzing. Please keep this in mind:

Without risk, there is no growth or energy; however, without support, risk becomes recklessness.

In the territory in-between we can grow, thrive, and find pleasure. This place between too much support or sensation and too little is called the Resilient Edge of Resistance.

My late teaching partner, Chester Mainard, a sublime instructor of healing and erotic touch, coined the phrase "Resilient Edge of Resistance." He initially created the term to describe the ideal way to touch.

Try this: Place your hand on your lower arm very lightly. Don't apply any pressure. Notice what this feels like. Now massage your arm, applying increasingly more pressure. Stop at the point where the massage becomes painful. Notice what that feels like. Now, lighten your touch until you feel the point at which your arm yields to your touch but doesn't shrink away from it. That touch, perfectly placed between too much and too little, is the Resilient Edge of Resistance.

The Resilient Edge of Resistance applies to more than just touch. It also applies to the emotional body. Remember the last time you shared with a friend a really challenging problem you were having? How did your friend respond? Did they dispassionately offer platitudes, looking as though they wished they were somewhere else? Did they leap in with dozens of suggestions and try to solve the problem for you? Or did they offer a balanced combination of attentive listening, appropriate questions, and a couple of new ways that you might look at your situation? When people do not meet our level of emotional involvement in a situation, we feel frustrated or discouraged. When they try to take over, we feel overwhelmed or powerless. When they respond with just the right form of empathy—a response that meets our emotional Resilient Edge of Resistance—we feel heard, safe, and supported.

This is the kind of safety we want to create as we anticipate entering into new erotic and ecstatic waters. We want to be sufficiently supported to take a risk. The Resilient Edge of Resistance occurs at different depths in different situations for each individual. Safety—and what creates it—is a highly individual choice. Some people, for example, feel more comfortable learning new erotic skills with a group in a workshop setting. Others could not even imagine learning these skills in anything other than a private session with only their partner and a teacher present.

The principle of a sufficient support to take a risk applies to relationships. Our most successful and exciting relationships are those in which we are both supported and challenged. Whether it's your life partner, the director of a play you're performing in, the editor of the book you're writing, your coach, or your boss, the relationships we treasure and remember are those in which we feel closest to a perfect balance of challenge and support, risk and reward.

Those of us who frequently take erotic risks, and/or lead others in workshops where they learn to do the same, strive to create safe containers for erotic explorations. A new safe container must be constructed for each new encounter. We spend a lot of time talking about, thinking about, and creating safe space. In one of my recent professional training programs, my colleague, Swedish sex educator Carl Johan Rehbinder, suggested we stop using the phrase "safe space" and instead, think of the spaces we create for erotic and ecstatic explorations as "magic rooms." It quickly dawned on everyone in the group how this simple change of phrase more perfectly met and expressed the Resilient Edge of Resistance we were looking for in our workshop spaces. We want the spaces we play and pray and make love in to be safe. But more than safety—we want *magic*—and that must include room for risk to take its appropriate place.

I asked my Facebook and Twitter focus group—many of whom create "magic rooms" themselves: If you were going to take an erotic risk—try something new or go somewhere you have not been before—what would you need in place to feel safe enough to do it?

The rest of this chapter is dedicated to the discussion of these elements, many of which I've distilled from the answers to my question on Facebook. Open to a new page in your notebook. As you read through these elements of safety, take note how each might or might not make you feel safe.

Physical and Environmental Safety

As Chester often said, "In order to feel emotionally safe, we must first know we are physically safe." Physical safety—the most basic form of safety—applies to both your physical body and the physical location of your "magic room." Let's start with your body.

Your Body

First and most important to know, sex should not hurt—unless you want it to, of course. Some people do like their sex rough. They love sensations so intense that other people would call them painful. This kind of consensual, carefully delivered pain is not the kind of pain I'm talking about. I'm talking about unwanted, unpleasant pain. Pain during sex is more common than people admit and it affects both men and women. It can be caused by a variety of physical or psychological factors. Often the problem is easily treatable but people feel too embarrassed to ask for help. Recent studies suggest that more than 60 percent of women report current or previous episodes of pain during sex. Fewer than half of these women discussed this pain with their doctors.

This means a significant percentage of people are putting up with pain until it either becomes unbearable or they stop having sex because of it. Here is a list of some of the most common causes of pain during sex. A longer discussion on the symptoms, causes, and treatments appear in Afterglow A on page 231.

For women (or people of any gender with a vulva and a vagina):

- Vaginal dryness

- Inflammation of the tissue of the vulva

- Vaginismus (a condition in which the muscles around the opening of the vagina spasm shut)

- Vaginal scarring

- Deeper cervical or pelvic pain

For men (or people of any gender with a penis and testicles):

- Prostatitis (an inflammation or infection of the prostate gland)

- Epididymitis (a swelling of the tube that connects the testicle with the vas deferens)

- Peyronie's disease (essentially, arthritis of the penis)

- Psoriasis and dermatitis

- Phimosis and paraphimosis (conditions in which the foreskin is too tight to be completely retracted over the head of the penis, or in which the foreskin is stuck behind the head of the penis and can't be pulled forward)

For people of all genders:

- Urinary tract infections, yeast infections

- Chlamydia, genital warts, gonorrhea, hepatitis, herpes, HIV, molluscum contagiosum (aka MC or water warts), scabies, syphilis, thrush, and trichomoniasis are just a few of the sexually transmitted diseases that can cause pain.

- Sexual pain is not limited to the genitals. Some people avoid anal sex because they fear that it will hurt, and when performed incorrectly, it can. Although existing hemorrhoids or anal fissures (tears) would certainly make anal sex painful, more often pain during anal sex is a sign that it's being performed incorrectly. The receiver may be too tense, the giver may be pushing too hard, there might not be enough lubricant, or the penis or toy may be too large. Using fingers, smaller toys, copious amount of lube, and proceeding very slowly will usually make the experience pleasurable and pain-free.

The first step in alleviating any physical pain you're having during sex is to determine if there is a body-level cause that needs help or treatment. And yes, pain during sex may simply be a sign that you need to slow down and use more lube. However, any occurrence of sexual pain that is not easily alleviated by one or both of these methods should be taken seriously and investigated by a medical professional.

Safer Sex: Practicing safer sex is the most fundamental and crucial physical safety precaution you can take. Safer sex means sexual activity with no exchange of bodily fluids. Which bodily fluids? These: ejaculate (male or female), blood (including menstrual blood), vaginal secretions, urine, feces, and the discharges from sores caused by sexually transmitted infections. "No exchange" means that none of the bodily fluids of one partner ever gets into the vagina, penis, anus, mouth, eyes, nose, or open skin wounds of another.

Safer-sex protocol is necessary when either you or your partner has any sexually transmitted infections (STI), including—and this is the important part—*when you aren't sure.* Unless you are in a strictly monogamous relationship with someone whose HIV/STI status you are certain of, you need to know about and practice safer sex.

You may be thinking that safer sex is something you—for whatever reason—don't have to worry about. Perhaps you have been with the same partner for years. Or perhaps your only sex partner is yourself right now. Nevertheless, please read the safer-sex guidelines in Afterglow B on page 234. As you go further into ecstatic experiences you may find that you want to explore something new. That new something or someone may present the need to make a new decision about safer sex.

The time to make safer-sex decisions is before you take your clothes off.

Everyone should have a basic safer-sex supply kit within easy reach. You don't need a lot of stuff to play safely. You can put a safer-sex kit together with a few essential basics, such as condoms; lubricants; latex, vinyl, or nitrile gloves; plastic wrap; and hand sanitizer. Advanced or esoteric ecstatic practices require additional supplies.

Environmental Safety

Once you have established safety protocol for your physical body, extend this sense of safety to your physical environment. What do you need to create your magic room?

Perhaps you always wanted to make love outdoors in a public space. That's a juicy and not uncommon fantasy. However, you wouldn't want to try it on the top of a hill during a massive thunderstorm. Think about it: Does your environment support your intentions? Are safer-sex supplies available? If your desire requires toys or equipment, are those toys and equipment available and in good condition? If your fantasy involves handcuffs, do you know where the key is?

Keep your rituals appropriate to your physical surroundings and plan ahead. Does your fantasy involve lots of noise or public exposure? Does it contain anything that could become a physical or legal risk? Erotic adventures are seldom ecstatic when interrupted by the police, the fire department, or a trip to the emergency room.

Physical safety goes beyond avoiding situations in which you could be physically harmed and extends into the sensual elements of your environment that make you feel emotionally safe. For example, what does comfort mean to *you?* For some people it might be the feel of wet grass. For others it's a huge stack of pillows on a feather bed. Which smells comfort you? Which turn you off? I have had to leave many a Tantric ritual where the air was ripe with the aroma of bananas and tropical fruit, which was a sensuous turn-on for most participants, but made me nauseous. And how about the lighting? Does it make you feel like a sex god or goddess, or does it reveal every physical flaw? How about the noise level or the choice of music? In my workshops I try to pick music to appeal to the greatest number of people, but occasionally I will pick something that is a complete turnoff to someone in the room.

C⋇Ɔ

*Take a few moments to write down a
few sensual elements that always make you
feel safe, centered, and special.*

C⋇Ɔ

How do you feel about crowds, groups, or the presence of other people? Some people delight in being erotic around other people. From a purely energetic standpoint, the more people you have raising erotic energy, the more intense the energy field. Group energy can be an ecstatic power source you can tap into. However, not everyone likes being erotic in public. Many of us have an inner exhibitionist and/or an inner voyeur of one sort or another, but playing in public is not everyone's cup of tea. For example, perhaps you would enjoy going to a sex club to watch a stripper perform, but never would consider actually stripping in public yourself. Or, perhaps you're more like my friend, Vicky, who became a burlesque performance artist. Vicky says, "I always feel much safer in front of a crowd than in the middle of one." Which one feels safer for you: would you rather watch or perform?

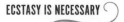

How do you feel about public vs. private sex?
When do you feel comfortable in a group?

There are some ecstatic experiences—such as trance dancing in a drum circle—that require a group in order to bring the ecstasy to its greatest expression. Dancing alone in your living room simply would not have the same effect.

Whatever your preferences now (and remember, they may change) simply make note of them. Keep in mind that different activities involve varying levels of risk and will require appropriate degrees of physical and environmental safety.

Choosing the Right Time

The timing of your erotic adventure is an important consideration from both a safety and an ecstasy-making point of view. First and foremost, don't plan an elaborate erotic adventure when you're exhausted or emotionally drained. Ecstatic adventuring requires endurance and mindfulness, none of which you'll have after handling a major crisis or at the end of an 60-hour workweek. Secondly, make sure you have *enough* time to do whatever it is you'd like to do.

Picture this: you and your partner have spent months creating a beautiful sexual ritual for yourselves. You're planning to start with a sensual bath, then move into the living room for some erotic massage in front of the fire, followed by some hot action in the kitchen, and ending with a grand finale in the bedroom. Because of the demands of your jobs and your family life, you've been putting this off for months. You finally decide that you're going to do your ritual this coming Saturday night—no matter what.

Saturday turns out to be a wildly busy day, filled with chores and commitments. Come Saturday night, you wind up with only two hours instead of the six you thought you were going to have. You proceed with your ritual anyway. Just as you have reached an intensely open and intimate state in front of the fire, your daughter comes home early from a failed blind date. Suddenly you are yanked out of your altered state and slammed back to earthly reality with no transition time. Instead of feeling transformed, you feel angry, resentful, and emotionally injured.

Please make sure you have enough time to do what you want to do. Embarking on an erotic adventure means having enough time to process the results, be they emotional revelations, physical releases, or transcendental experiences.

A good rule if you're planning to try something you've never tried before is to allow twice as much time as you think you'll need. This will give you plenty of time to set up, talk about things in advance, start slowly, and stop to rethink or renegotiate if you need to, with plenty of time left to decompress at the end.

Communication

Communication is required in all stages of erotic and ecstatic activity, but the nature and style of communication can vary widely. Later on we'll look at different styles of communicating and some effective ways to negotiate new erotic territory. Right now I'd simply like you to think about what kind of communication you need to give and receive in sexual situations in order to feel safe. Here are a few examples.

Some people need to feel heard. Others need to be reassured. Some want dirty talk—or to be told how gorgeous and hot they are. Some need encouragement. Some people go into a wordless trance and only want to hear essential spoken communication. How much communication do you need and when do you need it most—before, during, or after an erotic encounter?

Review the needs exercise in Chapter 2 to see what is most important for you when it comes to communication. Different erotic activities demand different communication. For example, your most important communication needs on a day-to-day

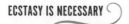

basis might be to be able to trust in another's word, commitment, and adherence to agreements. However, if you wanted to engage in a role-playing scene in which you are a naughty five-year-old, your needs might be different. You may need a partner with the communication skills to give you a creative scenario, emotional support, and unconditional acceptance of whatever feelings might arise.

If you're experimenting with a new sex toy, a lighthearted, playful, humorous tone might be most appropriate. In the scene involving your inner naughty five-year-old, a confident, dominant, and even demanding tone may be required to make your "little girl" feel safe and turned on.

We'll explore communication more thoroughly in Chapter 6. Let's move on to the next element in creating erotic safety.

Consciousness/Mindfulness

One of the most essential ingredients of an ecstatic experience is mindfulness. Mindfulness, or consciousness, is simply staying in each present moment and putting your attention on your intention. For example, if your intention is to give your partner exquisite oral sex, you'll go totally into the taste, texture, touch, and smells of your partner's delicious genitals. If you're practicing Tantra, you'll go totally into the breath, the shared energy, and the gaze of your partner's eyes.

Mindfulness transforms sex into a passionate active meditation. And like meditation, it requires some practice, and an ongoing dedication to staying focused. Mindfulness is the ultimate safety precaution. If you are totally present in each and every successive moment you will always be able to find safety.

Consent

There is a rule by which people in the BDSM (Bondage/Discipline, Dominance/Submission, Sadomasochism) communities play. It's called safe, sane, and consensual. Safe means that precautions are taken to keep everyone involved safe from physical harm. Sane means that the players are not under the influence of drugs or alcohol, and are not doing anything mean or malicious, and that everyone's emotional and mental safety are being cared for. Consensual means that everyone participating is doing so because they want to. No coercion of any kind is taking place and neither partner is doing anything to the other without their consent.

The cornerstone of your erotic safety is consent. Consent is not something that you give once, assuming it will apply to every aspect of every activity that follows. Nor does the consent you gave last night automatically apply to tonight. Let's say that you've always had a fantasy of being tied up and ravished by a stranger. You and your partner agree that it would be exciting to play out this scenario. You're a little nervous about being restrained, but that's part of the turn-on. So far so good. Your partner (who has done sufficient research on safe ways to tie you to the bed without cutting off your circulation) finishes tying you up and begins to ravish you. At first it's fun and hot and a huge turn-on. Then suddenly you look into your partner's eyes and all you can see are the eyes of the uncle who molested you when you were 14. Suddenly this isn't fun anymore—it's horrible. What do you do? You withdraw your consent by using your safeword.

A safeword is a word or a signal that communicates that you wish a scene to stop when it has become too challenging physically or emotionally. You choose this word or signal before you begin to play. Select a word that would not normally come up in the course of an actual erotic scene. The most common safewords are based on a traffic light model: Green for go, yellow for slow down, and red for stop. With a safeword in place, you can scream "No, no no!" or "Stop, you evil beast!" as much you like and the delicious ravishment you're enjoying continues. However, if you say "Red!" your partner immediately steps out of role, unties you, and helps you through whatever difficult emotions have just arisen. This is consensual play.

You may never choose to consent to this particular role-play scene again. Or, you may stop for a little while until you feel safe again, and then continue with this scene or another one. You may even find that playing out a hot-but-challenging scene is an empowering way to clear out old trauma. It's all up to you.

In the next chapter—Good Boundaries Make Good Lovers, I'll talk about the deeper meanings of the words *yes, no,* and *maybe.* For now, it's important to understand that consent does not mean being talked into something that you really don't want to do. Consent is not a maybe. Consent means yes—and preferably, an enthusiastic yes.

Escape Strategy

A safeword is only one form of escape strategy. You can create any form of verbal or nonverbal signal to communicate that you want to stop. Knowing that you can safely stop in the middle of an erotic adventure provides a lot of security. Strangely enough, with the exception of a safeword, people often do not put enough time and attention in planning an escape strategy. It seems that we fear that we will offend our partners if we discuss the possibility of our erotic adventure not working out.

An escape strategy is a form of communication—or, more precisely, *permission to communicate*—that something difficult is going on for you. It doesn't necessarily mean your partner did anything wrong. It just means that you are experiencing something that requires you to make a new decision about this particular erotic or ecstatic activity. Escape strategies are erotically supportive because they give everyone participating permission and encouragement to go totally into their experience, knowing that if they hit a rocky emotional place they can stop and get comfort or support with no judgment.

Escape strategies are applicable to emotional, physical, and social situations. They can be as simple as, "I want to try anal sex, but if I don't like it can we just stop and do something else?" Or if you are attending your first swingers' sex party with your partner, you can have a signal, a code phrase, or an arranged meeting time to tell your partner if you want to leave. Or if you're playing with bondage, you will definitely want to have a pair of safety scissors close at hand.

It is in the moments when you need to employ your escape strategy that you may find unimagined amounts of love and intimacy. Some of the most intense and rewarding experiences happen when your plan goes "wrong" and you find yourself in an unexplored land. That's when the empathy and compassion you receive from your partner(s) may create a peak ecstatic experience.

Right Mind-set

An important question to ask yourself is: Am I in the right frame of mind to take an erotic risk? Being in one's right mind is relative. Trying a new sex position after drinking one glass of wine too many is a relatively small risk, provided no other risks (such as trying this new position on the wing of a moving aircraft) are in place. However, trying mummification for the first time with a new partner on the evening following your mother's funeral may not be the safest and sanest choice. People are frequently tempted to take more extreme risks during intensely emotional times.

In a similar vein, are you on any medications or recreational substances that could alter the way you process sensation or emotion? Remember that the "sane" in safe, sane, and consensual does not just apply to your normal frame of mind—it applies to your actual state of mind in the present moment. Your state of mind can be altered by emotional turbulence in your life, as well as by drugs and alcohol.

Recently I passed through several years when it seemed like everyone I loved was either sick or dying. I felt levels of grief and stress so intense that it was often like being in an altered state. During that time I was very careful about who I invited on erotic dates, and how I played. I always made sure that any potential partner understood that I was likely to have an illogical or larger-than-typical reaction to anything we did. Nearly every time I raised any erotic energy I would have a huge crygasm or screamgasm. Instead of keeping a box of tissues within easy reach—I had a roll of paper towels. But because my partners understood that I was walking an emotional edge, they were able to help me release a lot of the pain and anguish I was feeling. I always felt "saner" after these sessions.

So, if you are not sure whether you're up for a potentially intense erotic experience, but you feel inclined to go ahead anyway, make sure you are with the right partner (see page 81) and make sure that your partner knows that you are in a fragile condition.

No Expectations

Some of my favorite words of wisdom are:

> *"Make no judgments, make no comparisons,*
> *and release your need to understand."*

Judging, comparing, and trying to figure something out—these almost always yank me out of the present moment. Just as soon as I jump into the past (comparing this event to something I have previously experienced) or future (by judging what it's going to be like or obsessing over how it's going to work), I am likely to scare myself silly with negative expectations, or intimidate myself with positive ones. As I tell my students in my breath and energy orgasm workshops, the most difficult part of learning how to have a breath and energy orgasm is learning how to release your expectations. If you expect to blast off into the center of the universe where the Goddess will share the secret of life with you, you're probably setting yourself up for disappointment. Similarly, if you assume that you'll never be able to have a breath and energy orgasm—that everyone else is going to have a great time and you will be lying on the floor like a lump, you are also setting yourself up for failure. I recommend an attitude similar to, "What the hell. I'm here anyway. I may as well lie down, breathe, and see what happens."

The Right Partner(s)

Just because someone looks really hot, or is rumored to be a Tantric guru, does not mean they are right—or safe—for you. And—just because you have been with someone for a decade and they know you better than anyone else, does not necessarily make them the right partner to accompany you on the next erotic/ecstatic adventure you want to take.

When you ask the question, "What kind of partner do I need to feel safe enough to take an erotic risk?" the answer might be your primary partner, if that's who you feel safest with when you think about exploring a new erotic or ecstatic territory. Or, it might be someone else—possibly a stranger or even a professional—who has the physical and emotional skills to take you to a new level of experience or understanding of the particular ecstatic risk you wish to take.

This, of course, raises the issue of monogamy and non-monogamy. What if you are in a monogamous relationship and your partner has no interest in exploring a particular erotic activity that you feel compelled to explore? Erotic explorers—whether experienced or just starting out—learn to apply the same level of consciousness to the co-creation of their relationships as they do to the creation of their ecstatic adventures. This means taking the time and making the effort to *choose* the level of emotional and/or sexual fidelity you want in your relationship, rather than letting the form of your relationship dictate the level of your emotional and/or sexual fidelity.

Some people think that monogamy is the natural state of human coupling. Others believe that monogamy is simply an act of social conditioning, and that we'd all be non-monogamous if we could break the binds of our monogamous upbringings. The reality of the situation is more complex than either of these positions. Judith Stacey, a New York University sociologist quoted in an article in the *New York Times Magazine*, states, "Neither monogamy nor polygamy is humankind's sole natural state . . . Monogamy is not natural, non-monogamy is not natural. Variation is what's natural."

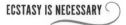

The subject of monogamy has been subjected to the same kind of binary thinking that has plagued the subject of gender. Just as we have come to understand gender as a spectrum, with most people falling somewhere in between the poles of completely male and totally female, fidelity also presents a panorama of choices. Monogamy is the right choice for some people. Other people—with the right partners and under the right circumstances—can be happy in various types of non-monogamous relationships. Other people are non-monogamous by nature and choice.

The issue is not whether monogamy is right or wrong, but whether it is appropriate for *you*. Monogamy is a choice—not the default, as my friend Betty Herbert eloquently explains in her book, *The 52 Seductions*, a memoir about how she and her husband made a pact to seduce each other once a week for a year.

> Monogamy isn't just one, dead choice. It is a daily, hourly choice that should be made in full acceptance of the other choices available. It should be a conscious choice made by two people, rather than a bland acceptance of "the done thing." If we fall into monogamy by default and never question it again, it will die. The compact can be broken by secret infidelities, but it can equally be broken by withdrawing love and affection. Taken in this way, monogamy is a radical choice among many rather than a bland following of convention. It is not for everyone, and no one should imply otherwise. But for me, it's just right.

Dan Savage, the nationally known sex advice columnist for *The Stranger* in Seattle professes to be "monogamish." He is in a long-term relationship that is mostly monogamous, but allows for what he terms "permissible infidelities." My friends Chris and Pat consider their relationship to be their spiritual practice. They describe themselves as a pair-bonded, non-monogamous, devoted, married couple. When they have sex with someone else, they usually—but not always—prefer to do it together. In all these cases, the choice to be monogamous or not—as well as *how* each choice would work—was made with care and consciousness.

There is a myth that non-monogamy is a callous, promiscuous, free-for-all in which everyone is bound to get hurt. Nothing could be further from the truth. Making conscious non-monogamy work is just as possible—and every bit as complicated—as making monogamy work. Ecstatic relationships are characterized by unconditional acceptance and authenticity. Creating ecstatic relationships requires integrity.

As Judith Stacey says, "What integrity means for me is we shouldn't impose a single vow of monogamy as a superior standard for all relationships," Stacey said. "Intimate partners should decide the vows you want to make. Work out terms of what your commitments are, and be on same page."

Do you need or expect sexual fidelity in your relationships? What is sexual fidelity—for you? For example, is it okay if your partner flirts with someone at a bar? Is it okay if they participate in a sexual exchange limited to text messaging? Would it be okay with you if they kissed someone else? How about emotional fidelity? Would you be comfortable with your partner enjoying a deeply emotional relationship with someone else so long as they remained sexually faithful to you? How would you feel if they wanted to see a professional sex worker? Or be sexual within the context of a sex education workshop?

My client, Sandra, came to me because she was desperate to explore her sexuality as part of a spiritual and emotional reawakening she was experiencing during perimenopause. She had married at age 32, having had little sexual experience prior to her marriage. Her husband was not at all open-minded about any of her new sexual and spiritual interests. He wouldn't accompany her to the Tantra workshop she wanted to attend, and he had no interest in experimenting with anything new at home.

Sandra was so eager for growth she felt like she was going to explode. She wanted to try *everything*, and she wanted it *now*. She had had an "emotional" affair a few months before, and was concerned that she would soon be in a full-blown affair—if not several—if she did not find a way to get her new needs met. Her husband had no objection to her personal development work thus far, but she was not sure how he'd feel about it if it included actual sexual contact.

We created a plan for Sandra that began with workshops where she could exchange sexual energy—but not explicit touch—with multiple partners. This gave her an experience of, and a vocabulary for, expanded ecstatic and erotic states. When she was able to let her intense sexual energy start to flow, her desire to do anything and everything with anyone started to subside. She was able to talk to her husband more articulately about what she needed. They agreed that he was not the person to accompany her down this particular path, but he had no objection to her participating in the next level of workshops—women-only workshops that did include erotic touch.

Little by little, and conscious step by conscious step, Sandra was able to find partners and practitioners that were able to meet her needs without terrifying her husband. Her marriage not only survived, but thrived.

Opening up an existing relationship to something other than monogamy requires patience, love, devotion and skill. For a list of resources to help you navigate these waters, see Afterglow C on page 239.

Ecstatic risk-taking—and all I mean by "risk" is the courage to take the next logical step in your erotic evolution—requires a partner(s) who shares your values and can meet your needs. Not every person can meet all your needs, nor will anyone share *all* your values in every area of your life. If your husband hates "chick flicks," for example, you'd ask a friend to accompany you to the latest romantic comedy, right? Why should erotic/ecstatic activities be any different?

Many people are more comfortable taking an erotic risk with people they do not know rather than with their partner, or with friends. If that is true for you, please don't think you are strange or abnormal. Besides, even if you have the world's most perfect partner in every respect, they may not be the right person to take that particular risk with at this particular time. Here's an example of that. Say you want to dance yourself into an ecstatic trance. You may need to find someone other than your primary partner who is about to schedule a knee replacement. Or, say your partner is obsessed with meeting a deadline for a huge project at work. The pagan faerie gathering that means so much to you might be completely off their radar. Find friends who share your curiosity and your passions. You can invite a platonic friend to partner with you at sex workshops. A majority of sex workshops do not involve nudity or explicit erotic touch. Simply find out in advance what is expected.

CXO

Take a moment to think about the people in your life with whom you might like to explore ecstatic experiences. Who is the right partner for you? For which activity(ies)?

CXO

Emotional Safety

All ecstatic experiences involve a degree of emotional risk. For some, the greater the risk, the greater the payoff. Others prefer a more conservative approach.

When deciding how much emotional risk you can tolerate, remember that if an erotic situation presents no risk at all, there will be little or no energy—and therefore little or no ecstasy—generated. If there is too much emotional risk, you'll be paralyzed with fear, and surely that leaves no energy for ecstasy. So, just how safe do you really want to be?

For optimal pleasure, you'll want safety and risk to meet at your resilient edge of emotional resistance—the place where you feel sufficiently and consistently supported to take a risk. This is highly individual and ever-shifting territory. A good place to start is by looking over your list of needs. There are, predictably, several basic categories of emotional safety that most people feel they need to have in place before they can take erotic or emotional risks.

The first is trust. For most of us, this means trust in one's partner or partners, but it can also extend to a group, or to an event.

We need to trust that we will not be embarrassed, humiliated, or hurt—before, during, or after an erotic encounter. This kind of trust is so essential to an ecstatic encounter and so basic to the foundation of intimacy that when this type of trust is violated it is usually experienced as the very worst form of betrayal.

Another key piece of emotional safety is believing that whatever you want to do is normal and okay. Although a certain level of naughtiness can be part of a turn-on, we need to feel that whatever we're doing is within the parameters of acceptability in at least one of our communities. For example, sex before marriage may be considered wrong in the religious community you grew up in. But if that religious community is not your primary social group now—and premarital sex is considered not only normal, but assumed in your social circles—you will probably feel perfectly safe having sex with your romantic partner. On the other hand, if you are a 20-something heterosexual man, and all your friends constantly joke and tease each other about how "gay" anal sex is, you may feel apprehensive about trying it, even with your long-time girlfriend. (This is called internalized homophobia.) Later on, I'll discuss how to find your new "normal" by changing your thinking and by receiving support from others.

"Just the right amount" of desire is an urban myth. We don't know what it is, but we suspect we are somehow out of its range. It's painful to feel left out, broken, and/or ashamed for a lack of desire, for too much desire, or for a desire for unusual things.

CXO

Have you ever felt this way? When? For what reason?

CXO

One of the places where it can be the hardest to find emotional support and safety is for a person's decision not to be sexual. You can be ecstatic on a regular basis and completely sex-positive (which simply means having a positive relationship to sexuality) and not be sexually active yourself. People who choose not to express their ecstatic selves in genital sex are becoming a more visible minority. Many asexual people simply don't experience sexual attraction. People who are celibate may feel attraction, but choose for whatever reason not to act on it. Some celibate people don't have sex with other people but continue to have sex with themselves. Others do not have sex at all. Still others identify as "stone," which is a sexual orientation in which someone's pleasure/desire is centered on another person's body and experience. "Stones" get their pleasure exclusively from giving others pleasure.

Give yourself permission to be exactly where you are on the spectrum of sexual desire. If you've been celibate for years and still have no physical desire for sex, let that be okay. Instead of beating yourself up about it, and ask, "What *does* turn me on?" It might be gardening, getting a massage, walking on the beach, or watching science-fiction movies.

EXERCISE: MY TOP TEN TURN-ONS IN LIFE

In your notebook, make a list of your top ten turn-ons in life. What do you really love to do? One of the items may be sex, but what are the other nine? When you finish your list ask yourself "When is the last time I gave myself any of the items on this list? Which item on the list feels the juiciest for me right now?" Make specific plans to give yourself one or more of your top ten turn-ons this week.

When you are able to give yourself the things that truly turn you on, you are likely to find that more and more things in life will turn you on. One of them may be sex. But remember, when we enter the Totality of Possibilities and think of all our erotic ecstatic experiences as sex, we are no longer limited or shamed by society and the media's rules and outdated morality. We are emotionally and ecstatically free.

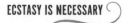

On the opposite end of the spectrum from asexuality and celibacy are the people who like sex "too much" or who like unusual activities. They have been told repeatedly that they are too loud, too intense, too sexual, too slutty, sick, or just plain weird. Judgments like this are often leveled by people who are simply envious of someone else's ability to travel well beyond traditionally accepted limits and boundaries. However, repeatedly hearing things like this can make you feel like you need to hold back your sexual expression for fear of being abandoned or judged once again. In order to feel safe enough to be your authentic sexual self you'll need to find communities in which your sexual expression is appreciated and applauded. I'll discuss that further in Chapter 5. But for now, please believe me when I say that it's possible to find a community of people who love like you do. A good way to find them is to love the way you love to love. That makes you a beacon for others who feel the same way.

Refuse to dwell on the question "Is this normal?" If you're feeling turned on by something, you can count on the fact that so are at least thousands, if not hundreds of thousands, of others. Replace "Is this feeling/attraction/desire/activity normal?" with "What about this could be fun?" "What about this could be liberating?" "What about this could be ecstatic?"

Exercise: Abnormal?

In your journal, or on a separate piece of paper, write down some of the things that you have done or imagined doing that you think are "not normal," "deviant" or "sick."

Only when you have completed this, look on the bottom of page 89 for the next instruction.

Having the Right Information/Education

One of the biggest concerns around taking any new sort of ecstatic risk is the fear of doing it wrong and/or looking stupid. In most cases having enough of the right information can easily allay these fears.

The lack of basic sex education in our culture is appalling. As I have previously mentioned, as adults we have to make a concerted effort to find the information we need in order to continue to grow as erotic beings. If you have been too ashamed and embarrassed to ask your friends or your doctor for some piece of sexual information, please know that you are not alone. I can prove it.

My colleague Marcelle Pick is the co-founder of www.womentowomen.com, a website and clinical practice dedicated to women's health. Women to Women offers help to over five million women a year. A large percentage of these women are seeking information about sexuality and/or sexual health. I asked Marcelle about women's needs for sexual information. Here are the questions Marcelle hears most frequently:

- I've lost my sex drive—where did it go?

- Sex isn't as comfortable as it used to be—what can I do?

- I'd like my partner to be more . . . creative. How do I start that conversation?

- Are sex toys okay to use?

- My partner just doesn't seem to be interested anymore—what can I do?

- My libido just doesn't match my partner's. What do I do?

- I don't have any desire to have sex. Is this normal?

- I've never had oral sex—but I'd like to learn more—can you recommend a site?

- I'm newly single and can't even think about sex with someone new. Help!

Now, imagine this is not your list, but your best friend's list. How abnormal, sick, or deviant do you think these things are now?

- My partner and I want sex at different times—how do we balance things out?

- I need more foreplay. It takes me a while to "warm up." Are other people like this?

- My partner wants to have anal sex—is it safe?

- How do I have an orgasm?

- How can I help my husband put off his orgasm?

How many of these questions can you relate to? How many of these questions, or similar ones, would you like to receive answers to? What other questions have you always wanted answers to?

You may need to look no further than the Internet, a good book, or a sex education video to find out all you need to know about subjects such as oral sex, anal sex, orgasm, or sex toys. However, if you'd like to practice Tantra, or learn Gabrielle Roth's 5Rhythms movement meditation practice, or learn how to put someone in rope bondage and suspend them in the air, you'll really need hands-on instruction. Take a workshop. Not only will you learn the skills more efficiently, you will also meet members of a new tribe who can encourage and support you in your new adventure.

There are more and more workshops and erotic education events happening in smaller cities and towns worldwide. However, if you're serious about pursuing advanced erotic arts, be prepared to travel occasionally, especially if you don't live in or near a major metropolis. Budgeting money for travel to events for advanced ecstatic experiences may turn out to become one of your favorite financial priorities. It has certainly made a world of difference for me.

Remember, you do not have to know everything there is to know about sex. You just have to know enough to do what you want to do. How do you know you've found the right answers to your questions? Check out several sources. Get more than one opinion. Try it for yourself. Ultimately, the only right answer is the one that works for you.

☙❧

Think of a curiosity you have about sex.
Google it. Find out more about it.

☙❧

Breathe

I have left the most important key to erotic safety and sanity for last. Breath is your single most powerful tool for physical, emotional, and spiritual transformation. Yet, most of us breathe barely enough to stay alive—it's simply a physical reality in our culture. Changing the way you breathe produces a perceptible change in consciousness and an equally perceptible change in the way you feel—that's also a physical reality. You can move from a state of fear or anxiety into a state of calm, relaxed awareness just by changing the way you breathe. But it's not all about learning new ways to breathe. It's also about learning to *remember* to breathe.

I have been using my breath both to calm myself down and to blast myself into extended orgasmic states for years. I am on quite intimate terms with my breath. Yet, I must admit that when I am upset or freaked out, I also forget to breathe. When that happens, the last thing I need is someone telling me to just breathe and be in the moment. If that single piece of advice were enough, I'd be in a permanent state of nirvana by now. What I can always use are a few practical hints on how to remember to breathe myself into the safety of the present moment on a regular basis.

Here are a few simple things to remember about breath. Breathing in and out through your nose is relaxing, especially if you make your exhale longer than your inhale. When we are upset, we either stop breathing, or we tend to breathe in and out through our mouths with shallow, fast gulps of air, often forcing the exhale. This kind of breathing can make us even more anxious and irritable, because when we breathe out too much carbon dioxide it causes an imbalance in the acid–base balance of the blood. When the amount of carbon dioxide in our blood falls below a critical point, the brain flips a switch and we stop breathing. This increases our anxiety, and may even lead to a full-on panic attack.

Here's a tip to remember: all you have to do to calm yourself with your breath is to slow your breathing down and breathe gently in and out through your nose with an exhale that's longer than your inhale.

However, different ways of breathing do produce slightly different effects, as anyone with experience in pranayama yoga knows only too well. The state that I find the most useful and pleasant for entering into and coming out of ecstatic experiences is one of relaxed alive awareness. This means that you are feeling calm and relaxed, yet also awake and aware, easily able to keep your attention focused on the here and now.

Here are two breath-based exercises I use when I want to move from an anxious state into a state of relaxed alive awareness. Both of these breaths help to ignite my intuition, and allow me to find my center and my sense of inner safety.

Exercise: Bottom Breathing

Bottom Breathing is a gentle, easy way to calm you down and open up your senses. It's the ideal breath to use when you want to move out of the busy or stressful state of doing into the easy, relaxed awareness of being.

1. Sit on the floor with your legs crossed (or on a hard-backed chair with your feet flat on the floor) and your spine straight. With your hands, pull the fleshy part

of your buttocks aside so you are sitting on your sit bones. (Once you learn the breath you can do it in any position.)

2. Place your hands on your belly. Relax your belly. Just let it go. Let it be round in your hands. (Despite the culture's fascination with concave bellies, bellies are supposed to be at least slightly rounded.)

3. Begin by exhaling all the air out of your lungs.

4. Then, as you inhale, very gently push out on the anal sphincter. Imagine that your anus can "kiss" the floor or the seat of the chair.

5. On the exhale, don't do anything. Don't contract your anus, don't hold it, don't push. Do nothing. Just let go.

6. Repeat. Inhale: out with the anal sphincter, in with the air. Exhale: do nothing.

7. Keep going.

That's all there is to it. If you find it hard to focus on your anus, try focusing on your belly button—it's doing the same thing. As you breathe in, your belly button and your anus move outward. As you exhale, they return to their original position without any effort on your part.

This breath may take a little while to get used to, as we are not used to focusing on our anuses. Although it may seem a little odd, this is actually a very natural breath; it's just not one you usually do when you are awake. This is how you breathe when you are sleeping deeply. If you watch someone sleeping on their side or stomach, you will see their buttocks and belly button moving outward on the inhale and relaxing on the exhale.

What can you expect to feel from this breath? Many people feel a warm flush in their face as the breath releases the tension in

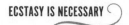

their bodies. Others report that it feels as though their whole body becomes a sense organ. Still others say it connects their upper and lower chakras. It produces a state of relaxed awareness quite unlike any other breath I have ever tried.

EXERCISE: COOK'S HOOK-UP

I learned this bioenergetic and kinesiology based exercise from author Cheryl Richardson and have been using it ever since. It's a wonderfully effective change-of-state exercise when you're feeling scattered, frazzled, anxious, or out of control.

1. Cross left ankle over right.

2. Extend both arms in front of you, with your hands back to back.

3. Cross your right hand over your left and clasp hands, fingers interlocked.

4. Bend your elbows so that your clasped hands turn under and in, toward your body, like a pretzel. Rest your clasped hands against your heart.

5. Place the tip of your tongue on the roof of your mouth, just behind your teeth. Inhale through your nose. Let your tongue relax down as you exhale through your mouth.

6. Gently hold this pose, gently, and continue the breathing for 1 to 2 minutes.

You can also practice this calm, centering exercise lying down.

You now have a better sense of what you need in order to feel safe enough to expand beyond where you are now into new ecstatic possibilities. Before we move on, please open your notebooks (or skim over this chapter from the beginning) and make note of the safety precautions and techniques that seem the most important to you. When you are done, *cross out all of them except the three that are truly the most important to you.* Here's why: if you try to implement every possible safety measure before you take an erotic or ecstatic risk, you'll never take a risk at all. The three safety measures you have decided are most necessary are more than enough to keep you safe as you take your next steps. If down the road a new erotic adventure brings up new fears and requires a new safety protocol, you can come back to your notebook and make new choices.

Now it's time to move on to the next step to creating transformative ecstatic adventures: setting good boundaries.

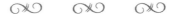

CHAPTER 4

Good Boundaries Make Good Lovers

Our boundaries help define us. They are the markers that show us where we stop and everything else begins. You've probably heard the phrase "good fences make good neighbors." Boundaries are to people what fences are to property—they mark what's mine from what's yours. Just how tall and impenetrable your fences need to be depends on factors such as where you live, who your neighbors are, the land conditions, and the preciousness of what's on your property. You might have a tall solid fence on one side of your property to keep your pet ostriches from escaping, or to protect a tender crop of clover from your neighbor's cows. At the front of your property you might have nothing more than a short decorative wall to keep people from parking on your front lawn. The best boundaries are permeable enough to let in things you want—such as friendly greetings from your neighbors—but keep out things you don't want—like those hungry cows.

Being clear about our own boundaries and respecting the boundaries of others is one of the most basic ways we build and demonstrate trust in any relationship. However, these are particularly important in intimate, ecstatic relationships. As I mentioned in previous chapters, ecstatic relationships are characterized by unconditional acceptance and authenticity. The essence of ecstatic experience is letting go into whatever happens—allowing yourself to become the experience. In order to do that, you need trust and a safe container—or magic room. In allowing yourself to become the experience, you also allow the experience to transform you—sometimes a little, sometimes a lot. After each of these changes, you may discover new needs and desires that require you to reset your boundaries. Like fences, personal boundaries need attention and repair, and occasional reconfiguration to accommodate a change in the landscape. Learning how to set, reset, and respect boundaries is a key element of ecstatic experience.

Boundaries are not just about who can do what to whom in relationships. You can have boundaries about food, your physical environment, behaviors, activities, people, or just about anything in the physical or nonphysical world. Some boundaries may seem random or silly, but are actually quite significant to our well-being. For example, I have strong boundaries around certain types of food. As I mentioned earlier, the mere smell of a banana, pineapple, mango, papaya, or any other kind of tropical fruit makes me nauseous. So does a mere whiff of Chinese food. People have suggested long and complicated explanations for this, ranging from speculations that I was forced to eat these foods as a child (I can't recall that happening) to a past life in a Chinese prisoner-of-war camp (I can't recall that either). I really don't care why I don't like these foods. I just don't want to smell them or eat them. I would never insist that everyone I know stop eating Chinese food or tropical fruit. I simply insist that they do so far away from me. I am more than happy to take a break from work or a workshop to allow my assistants or participants to go out for lunch where they can eat these foods. However, I do ask that they not bring them into my office or my workshop room.

We want to set limits around strong likes and dislikes. We certainly want to set a boundary any time we are being hurt in some way. We want to set limits about what we will and will not tolerate, both physically and emotionally. But some situations are less obvious and we may wonder if these require setting boundaries.

Recently, I went to the post office to mail a package. The line was long, as it usually is at this Harlem, New York City branch. I was the last one in the line. A woman came in huffing and puffing, carrying six heavy shopping bags from the local supermarket. She took one look at my unusual, vintage 1970s eyeglasses and launched into an enthusiastic rant about how wonderful they were. She told me she also had a fabulous pair of glasses and started digging in her large purse. *Uh-oh,* I thought. *Should I pretend to answer a phone call to get out of a long conversation with this person?* I took a breath and checked in. Was I feeling energized or drained by this woman? The answer surprised me: I was feeling somewhere between neutral and energized. So I said, "I'd love to see your glasses." They were indeed fabulous sunglasses—purple plaid Burberrys, to be exact. Our mutual admiration of our glasses led to a conversation about style in the 1960s, which revealed that we were the same age. We spent the rest of our long wait comparing our teenage years, hers in Harlem, mine in New England. It was a fascinating and inspiring conversation. We shared both fond memories and our future hopes and dreams. By the time we finally got to the service window we were disappointed the line had moved so quickly. We ended our encounter with a big hug.

It was a positively ecstatic chance meeting. I left the post office totally high. I had felt seen, heard, understood, and totally met by a woman whose name I had never learned. The anxieties I had been gnashing over on my way to the post office had vanished and been replaced by wonder at the magic of the synchronicities of life.

I could have easily put up a boundary and politely avoided talking to her. And that's probably what I would have done if I had made the decision with my brain instead of my energy meter.

My inner energy meter did not measure the character or sanity of the woman who liked my glasses. It did not make a judgment about her energy, as in "does this person have good energy or bad energy?" It measured only one variable: Am I feeling energized or drained in my interaction with this person? Does this situation provide me with an increase in energy, or is it sapping my energy?

This is the question I have learned to ask myself when I am unsure about the appropriateness of setting a boundary.

Ecstatic experiences require maximum exposure to people, places, and things that energize you, and minimal exposure to people, places, and things that drain your energy. The boundaries we set must be permeable enough to let in the love and solid enough to keep out the stress. Obviously, a Harlem post office is not a typical scene for an ecstatic experience. The boundary I chose to set in the post office was not about my new friend; instead, I made a conscious decision to ignore the impatience and the potential judgments of the people on line with us.

Ideally, we want to set up boundaries in advance, before we need them. However, we can't always evaluate whether a situation is going to be an energy gain or energy drain until we are faced with it. People resist setting boundaries for all sorts of other reasons. Many of us are just not very good at saying "no." When we set a boundary, we are in fact saying "No. I don't want to do that. I don't like that. Please stop." When we say "no" we risk disappointing people or making them angry. One of the primary reasons that people agree to sexual activities they don't really want to do is that they are afraid that if they don't, their lover will leave them or stop loving them. There are all sorts of risks involved when you set a boundary. You could be abandoned or embarrassed. Saying no might make you feel like you're being mean or selfish. You may worry that you are misreading the situation.

Boundary setting might be difficult if we weren't able to practice setting boundaries early on in our life. If you grew up in a home with emotionally unavailable parents, you may resist setting boundaries for fear of being as emotionally unavailable to others as your parents were to you. If you grew up in a home with extremely controlling parents who never permitted you to say no to them, you may have trouble saying no, or you may set overly strict boundaries and find yourself saying no to things that you would actually like to try. People who grew up in homes where there was domestic violence—whether or not they were abused themselves—often have the greatest trouble setting boundaries. Why? Because love, family, control, and violence are a combustible cocktail, and it can feel painful and dangerous—if not impossible—to try and find your limits.

In short, when we fail to set strong boundaries, it's almost always because we fear that something bad will happen to us if we clearly define who we are and what we like. However, setting clearly defined boundaries is vitally important for creating a safety net for ecstatic experiences. You can't take the risks you'll want and need without understanding your own boundaries and respecting other people's. Just as you must know what your needs are in order to get them met, you need to know what your boundaries are in order to set appropriate limits. Both ecstatic encounters and ecstatic relationships are highly creative processes and setting boundaries is a key component in all creative processes.

In one of my professional training programs I led a workshop in which I invited a group of soon-to-be sex coaches to envision their ideal practice. As part of this creative exercise, I asked them to tell me what their professional boundaries were. Sex coaching is a broad term that can define anyone from a sex surrogate who is likely to have actual physical sex with their clients, to a sex therapist whose license and code of ethics prohibits them from so much as touching a client. Clearly, boundaries must be considered when creating a practice as a sex professional.

The first time I asked participants to tell me their limits, the majority answered, "Well, I don't really have any boundaries. I'm pretty much willing to do whatever it takes to help my clients."

"Really?" I asked. "So if a client asked you to strangle them almost to the point of death for the purpose of achieving a more intense orgasm, would you do that?"

"Oh no!" they all exclaimed.

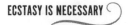

"Okay, we have found a boundary. What else won't you do?"

"Well," someone ventured, "I don't want to work past nine o'clock at night."

"Good, another boundary! How about intercourse? Are you willing to have sexual intercourse with your clients?" Most answered no; one or two needed to think about it. I kept asking them for more specific limits. By this time, everyone was perspiring and all were more than a little frustrated. This was clearly a very difficult exercise for the group. One participant, almost at her breaking point, asked, "Shouldn't we be envisioning what we do want instead of what we don't want? This is supposed to be a creative workshop for our new practices."

These sex coach trainees had spent over a year envisioning, practicing, and learning what they wanted for themselves and for their clients. Yet spending two hours getting clear on what they didn't want—what their boundaries were—was the hardest exercise of their training.

So don't be surprised or embarrassed if you have difficulty locating and communicating your boundaries. In the previous chapter we spent a great deal of time figuring out what we needed in order to feel safe in erotic and ecstatic experiences. Setting boundaries is simply another piece of the process of defining your needs and safety requirements. The time and effort you spend figuring out what you don't want eventually gets you a whole lot more of what you do want. When you create boundaries you're really creating the parameters of the magic room in which you will have infinite creativity and a Totality of Possibilities.

Boundary-Building Tools

Like fences, boundaries can be built from a variety of materials. Your most basic boundary is your skin. Your skin defines the outer boundary of your physical self. This physical boundary is how you first experienced yourself as separate from your mother, and then from the rest of the world. Victims of physical and sexual abuse often have a poor sense of boundaries because early in their lives they were taught that their most precious property—their bodies—didn't really belong to them. Others could invade their bodies and do whatever they wanted. The first boundaries we want to set are ones about who can touch us, how they can touch us, and when they can touch us.

When you were a small child, did you have an older relative who would grab you and hug and kiss you mercilessly whenever they saw you? Do you remember how much you hated it? Even though this relative adored you and thought they were expressing their unconditional love, they were in fact, violating your boundaries. I had an aunt who regularly mauled me in just this way. I remember my mother telling me that I could not protest or pull away. "That's just how Aunt Dell is. You'll hurt her feelings if you tell her to stop." To this day I will sometimes put up with touch with which I am slightly uncomfortable to avoid hurting someone's feelings. I still have trouble saying no.

Just say no. My good friend Dr. Mona Lisa Schulz and I were discussing boundaries. Dr. Mona Lisa is neuroscientist and a neuropsychiatrist. She's absolutely brilliant about all things brain- and emotion-related. When I asked Dr. Mona Lisa for her take on boundaries and sex, I expected a deep, scholarly, scientific, and profound answer. Instead the conversation went like this:

MLS: Shall we have Chinese food tonight?

BC: ML, you know I hate Chinese food.

MLS: Why?

BC: Why what?

MLS: Why do you hate Chinese food?

103

BC: Well, I don't know, I just do. Even the smell of it makes me sick . . .

MLS: But why? I don't think you've had the right kind of Chinese food.

BC: No, really. I have tried different of kinds of Chinese food. I hate it. It's nasty. It makes me physically sick.

MLS: I just don't think you're trying hard enough. I'm sure you could find something on the menu you could eat.

BC: No, ML, it's really nasty. I know lots of people like it, but I just really can't be around Chinese food.

MLS: When was last time you even tried any Chinese food? How do you know that this is even still true?

BC: Because the last time I ate Chinese food I was sick for days. . . .

By now I was anxious, confused, and desperate. I felt betrayed and more than a little crazy. I doubted myself. Perhaps there was something on a Chinese food menu that I could actually eat. Perhaps I was being too rigid about my dislike of Chinese food. I stared down at my hands and quietly shredded a Kleenex as I became more and more distraught. When I finally glanced up at Mona Lisa she was smiling mischievously. "Now," she said, "let's replace the words 'Chinese food' with the word for a sex act you don't like . . . Get it?"

We can all get confused and upset when someone challenges our boundaries. It can seem easier to just give in and try the Chinese food, or the sex. We think, "Perhaps it's selfish to withhold my time, my love, my energy, or my money, when someone else seems to need it or want it so badly. It might be easier to give in than to cope with the guilt. I'm just not good at saying no."

A friend of mine, sex educator Reid Mihalko, likes to play a "Just Say No" game in one of his sex and relationship workshops. You sit across from a partner. This partner asks if they can do something sensual or sexual with you—kiss you, for example. No matter what your feelings are about what they asked, you must say no. If they ask if you'd like a full-body massage with feathers and scented oils, you say no. If they ask if you'd like to be mummified in plastic wrap, you say no. If they offer to dip you in chocolate and lick it off, you still say no. Try this exercise. It is not only fun and funny, it's also quite intoxicating to feel the word "no" become both empowering and harmless.

Because the partner making the requests is certain that the answer is going to be no, they take absolutely no offense. Most people get very creative with their erotic requests when they know they are not going to be expected to follow through with it. The person saying no gets the reward of watching their partner smile and hearing them continue to offer more and more exotic and outrageous invitations. I urge you to try it. Keep in mind, if you hear something you really would like to try, you can always ask for it *after* the game ends.

Get some physical distance. One of the most effective ways to set a boundary is to put distance between you and what you don't like or want. You can leave the room, take a walk, or move across the country. Removing yourself physically from the situation will help give you a chance to reset your boundaries and find your emotional center.

Even if you cannot remove yourself permanently from a situation, you can still minimize your exposure. One of the best pieces of advice I received when I was coping with my two elderly parents who had become abusive toward each other was, "Get in, and get out." Meaning, I went to see them only as frequently as was necessary to oversee their care, and never stayed longer than one overnight. While I was there, I found numerous opportunities to get out of their house to go shopping or to eat. When I had to be with them for occasional longer periods, I stayed in a hotel. This way I could remain supportive of their needs, but avoid most of their attempts to drag me into the middle of their drama.

Excusing yourself to go to the bathroom or to return a phone call is another effective way to remove yourself from toxic situations, but there are situations where removing yourself from the scene is just not possible. In those cases, use your imagination and call in a natural element: imagine a big body of water between you and the toxic person or situation.

Here are a few more boundary-setting techniques.

Take a break. Have you ever become overwhelmed by a commitment you made to a person or a project? Has something that began as a romantic or exciting adventure turned into a time-consuming chore? Taking time off from a relationship or a project is a way of stopping the energy drain in some out-of-control aspect of your life. This does not mean that you have to permanently banish the person or the activity from your life. You just need some time away. Perhaps your 18-year-old really should live in a college dorm next year, and your favorite charity could continue to thrive if you weren't the chairperson of the fundraiser.

Get others to help. Sticking to our boundaries requires support. Have you ever broken up with someone and then desperately wanted to contact them, even though you knew it was a bad idea? Or made a decision to eliminate something from your diet, but felt your resolve weaken after a few days? What did you do? I have a list of friends and a therapist that I know I can count on for support when I feel this kind of boundary begin to dissolve. Simply talking to them is all I need to break the spell. I also rely on the Internet. Even if I need support in the middle of the night, chances are one of my friends on the other side of the world is up and checking her Facebook messages. One caveat about Internet support: keep private conversations private! This may seem obvious, but it's amazing the amount of damage that can occur when public posts are misinterpreted or read by the wrong people.

Get some emotional distance. Getting emotional distance in highly charged situations can be difficult. Our emotions may seem more powerful than our desire to set and maintain a healthy boundary. We may love someone who does not love us, or who treats us badly. We may fear that if we withdraw our love or emotional intimacy from an abusive relationship that we will be alone, or even be physically hurt. Getting emotional distance may require physical distance, taking time away from a person, and getting others to help. In addition, meditation, therapy, and other practices allow you to separate your higher self from your emotional self. Try observing your thoughts with detachment, as if they were clouds passing by in the sky.

Boundaries: Some Finer Points

The art of setting limits is finding the most effective ways to let in the greatest amount of love while blocking anything that feels like something other than love. Let's look at some of the more subtle aspects of setting appropriate boundaries, including how to decide when to set a boundary, around whom you can set boundaries, the role of intuition in setting limits, and how to adapt when situations change.

External vs. Internal Boundaries

We cannot put limits on what other people do. We can, however, limit our own exposure to people's behavior. If we can't bear the sound of honking freeway traffic, we can take a slower, scenic route to work or we can take the train. If we feel violated by violent movies, we don't have to watch them. We cannot expect frustrated people to stop honking, or expect Hollywood to stop making brutal movies. We can only control our exposure to the things that drain our energy. These are internal boundaries— choices we make to avoid certain things. The internal boundaries we set are just as important as the ones involving other people. This does not mean that we should become judgmental, cruel, self-disciplinarians. We can learn to say no lovingly—not only to our destructive desires and to desires that would be best fulfilled at another time—but to anything that significantly or regularly drains our energy.

Often when we set a boundary involving other people, we are asking them to do something differently when they are in direct contact with us, such as my request for participants not to eat bananas in my workshop room. Occasionally, we need to establish a boundary that asks others to behave differently, or to restrict certain behaviors even when they are not around us.

My friend Cecilia was married to a man who developed an obsession with Internet pornography. He spent countless hours glued to the computer, masturbating. Unsurprisingly, their sex life began to suffer. Not only was he less interested in Cecilia, when he did make love to her, he seemed to expect the "porn star experience"—he wanted her to behave in the exaggerated manner he was used to seeing on his computer screen. He had difficulty achieving orgasm without the same level of sexual overload to which he had become accustomed when he masturbated. Naturally, Cecilia felt unseen by her husband. Sex and all erotic touch became profoundly unsafe for her. She has since divorced her husband and is now interested in dating again. However, she still has a lot of fear about being touched sexually. She explains to potential lovers that she has a boundary: She will not enter into a relationship with any man who regularly masturbates to Internet porn. She does not expect them to forever abstain from all Internet porn. She simply will not be in relationship with anyone who watches it more than occasionally.

Cecilia realizes that her boundary places a condition on the private behavior of someone else. However, she is completely upfront about her boundary, so anyone who is uncomfortable with it simply does not have to date her a second time. The consensual nature of this agreement makes it work.

Hard Boundaries vs. Flexible Boundaries

In BDSM (Bondage/Discipline, Dominance/Submission, Sadomasochism) there is something called a Yes/No/Maybe list. The Yes/No/Maybe list is a long list of erotic activities—like a menu. Next to each choice you can check *yes* for "Sure! I'd love to," *no* for "I would absolutely never want to do that," or *maybe* for "I might consider that if circumstances were right." *No* would be considered a hard boundary; *maybe* is a flexible boundary. However, in this context, *maybe* always means *no* until or unless the person specifically states that their *maybe* has become a *yes*.

Remember my friend Reid's "Just Say No" exercise? Here is a variation that will help you learn to say no until your maybes have become yeses. This time, when your partner asks if they can do something sensual or sexual with you, you may answer yes or no. If you answer yes to your partner's request to kiss you on the nose, you get a kiss on the nose, right there and right then. If your partner once again asks if you would like them to give you a full-body massage with feathers and fragrant oils and you say yes, that's what you'll get right here and right now. But maybe you don't have time for that massage now. Or perhaps the room is a bit cold. Or perhaps you don't know your partner well enough yet. Or you may think, *Gee that would be so much nicer in my room after dinner tonight.* So, what's your answer? It's *no*, because *maybe* is always a *no . . . in the present moment.*

Think of all your *maybes* not as rejections, but as a source of delightful future possibilities. This is the proper use of flexible boundaries—when and if the timing and conditions are right, you'll be able to give your partner an enthusiastic *yes*.

The rule that maybe–means–no–unless–or–until–it–becomes–a–yes applies to far more than erotic touch. It applies to boundaries of all types. When people consistently and conscientiously respect our boundaries we may feel comfortable enough to relax some of them. This is a good thing, since when we are able to trust, we feel safe enough to take a risk. Taking risks is a key element in creating ecstatic experiences. I'll talk more about that in the next chapter. When people consistently violate our boundaries, we need to tighten those boundaries. We do this by creating consequences if the boundary is violated. For example:

- If you ever hit me again I will leave you.

- The next time you do not pay your share of the rent on time you will have to move out.

- You cannot call me in the middle of the night unless it is an emergency. If you do so again I will have to stop talking to you altogether.

- You know that I am perfectly okay with your other lovers. However, it is not okay for you to have sex with them in our bed. If you do so again, I will move out.

The challenging part of tightening boundaries is that you have to be prepared to actually follow through with the promised consequences if the boundary is violated. Consider how many lives might be saved if everyone who uttered "I will leave you if you ever hit me again" were to follow through with their promise the next time they were assaulted.

Different Boundaries for Different Folks

Just as your needs are different with different people, so are your boundaries different around different people. For example, you might be thrilled if one person offered to brush your hair, but horrified if another person did. It's perfectly okay to have different boundaries for different circumstances and different people—even if that makes other people angry. Some classic examples of the opposition you can face when you declare individualized boundaries are:

- You had sex with him. How come you won't have sex with me?

- You spent $300 on a gift for your mother and you won't loan me $200 so I can get my car fixed?!

- You spent all day last Sunday with her and her friends. Why can't you spend this Sunday with me?

Boundaries are not an egalitarian policy—your time, money, attention, and love do not have to be equally divided between everyone you know.

This, of course, brings up the question of how to stick to your boundaries when other people don't fully respect them. We will discuss this further in the chapter on communication, but suffice to say, you don't owe anyone a long explanation about your boundaries. You are not obligated to give them your childhood history. You don't have to share your therapist's opinion on the importance of your boundary. You don't have to promise to work on changing or eliminating this boundary. In fact, I heartily recommend you don't. When we engage in overly long or complicated defenses of our boundaries, we are likely to either jump off topic, invite debate, weaken our boundary, or step into judgments as a defense mechanism—just as I started to do when Mona Lisa challenged my boundary about Chinese food.

EXERCISE: DEFINE OR REFINE A BOUNDARY

In your notebook, describe a boundary that you a) need to set, or b) have set, but need to adjust, or c) have had violated. If this is a new boundary, list three boundary-building tools you will use to set your boundary and enforce it. If you've selected a boundary that has been violated and/or needs adjustment, describe how you'll strengthen it or change it. State the consequences you'll set if your boundary is violated. Or explain how you'll reset your yes, no, or maybe.

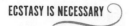

Privacy vs. Disclosure

Values and needs around privacy and disclosure vary widely across cultures and individuals. Within large extended families, it may be considered inappropriate, rude, and/or hurtful to withhold factual or emotional information from other family members. It may be equally inappropriate and even traitorous to share family secrets outside of the family. A clan's support system and survival is based upon everyone knowing everything going on within the clan, and keeping that information from outsiders. In these situations, family boundaries are prioritized over individual boundaries.

In smaller families made up of one or two parents and a couple of children, individual boundaries within the family may have a different value. Family members may agree to knock on doors before entering, be scrupulous about not listening to each other's phone conversations, and give each other a lot of "space." However, they may be quite open to sharing family "secrets" (such as quarrels or other domestic issues) with friends and in social situations.

Similarly, individuals have their own needs and expectations about privacy. In many cases, our privacy needs are paradoxical. We may be an exhibitionist in one area of our lives, and very private in another. For example, people who are consistently in the public eye are often manically private about their children, or may hire extensive security to keep the press away from a family wedding. If you have privacy needs that seem inconsistent, you are not unbalanced or inauthentic. It's actually normal and healthy.

In an age of ever-expanding social media outlets, many people are re-examining what they wish to keep private and what they want to make public. For people who use the Internet to find sex partners and make friends, this is of particular concern. How much do you post on a profile page that could be seen by anyone? It's no surprise people create false or altered identities. Pretending to be someone other than who they are may not simply be a desire to appear to be a better catch to a potential mate. I suspect it may also have something to do with the desire to keep some piece of the real self private until trust is established, either online or in person.

Erotic images posted on the web or "sexted" to a lover may circulate on the web forever. In the long run, this may be an important agent of social change. Years ago, tattoos were considered the mark of a dangerous, worthless, troublemaker, or at the very least, someone decidedly lower class. I remember my mother having nothing short of a breakdown when she found out I had pierced my ears. She was from an immigrant family and pierced ears were a sure sign of lowly, immigrant status. So perhaps having erotic pictures of oneself on the Internet may eventually be considered no more radical than having a couple of piercings and a tattoo. Perhaps when the vast majority of people are expressing their own unique erotic selves on the Internet, we will all be free to be more sexually authentic. But in the short-term, a lack of privacy boundaries online may cost you dearly.

Establishing your boundaries with regard to privacy is crucial for being able to establish intimacy when and where you want to. If you have no secrets—if everybody knows everything about you—how is one relationship more intimate than another? If everyone has access to your innermost thoughts and feelings, you risk being regularly drained by others. Remember, one of our best indicators of a healthy boundary is: "Am I feeling energized or drained? Does this situation provide me with an increase in energy, or is it sapping my energy?" It is up to you to establish who you choose to disclose what to. You may request and expect that your partner and your friends keep private whatever confidences you name—not only what *they* think should stay private.

Similarly, taking in too much information about other people is equally draining. When we are constantly receiving extraneous information about everyone we know, our energy is being pulled toward them and away from us. Have you ever read someone's personal post online and thought, *TMI! TMI! (Too much information!)* Similarly, haven't you known someone who can't resist gossiping and sharing absolutely everything that's going on with everybody else in their lives? Doesn't it make you fear an intimate emotional conversation with this person? On one hand, you want to make a connection that's only between the two of you. On the other, you wonder if tomorrow they will be telling everybody else everything you talked about. This is a particularly important boundary in non-monogamous relationships. It's important to be specific about how much of your personal news and information you want shared with your partner's other lovers, and how much you want to hear about their lives in return. It is up to you and your partner(s) to define what honesty, privacy, secrecy, and disclosure mean for you in the context of your relationship(s). The nature and degree of disclosure that works perfectly in one relationship may feel like secrecy—or too much information—in another.

Inner Guidance vs. Judgment

The process of establishing our boundaries requires us to make judgments. *Making a judgment is not the same thing as being judgmental.* We make appropriate and necessary judgments all the time. For example: It's cold outside so I better wear my warmest jacket. Or, I don't want to go mountain climbing because I am afraid of heights. Or, I don't want to hang out with that person because she's always mean to me. If we didn't make judgments we wouldn't survive very long.

One of the ways we make judgments is by using our intuition. Our intuitive guidance is like a radar system that is constantly tracking, even when our logical mind is focused elsewhere. Dozens of times a day our intuitive radar helps us avoid something inappropriate, uncomfortable, embarrassing, or dangerous. Some of us are more practiced at listening to and relying on our intuition than others.

When we listen to our intuition, we can make a judgment that allows us to form an opinion. Having an intuitive feeling about a situation helps us to navigate our way around it or through it. Having an opinion about something—whether it's a person, place, situation, or an idea—allows us to communicate in a focused way. Both opinions and intuitive feelings are fluid and can change as the person, place, situation, or idea changes.

Judgmental statements, on the other hand, are final assessments about whether something or someone is inherently good or bad. Judgments stop the conversation, whereas opinions invite dialogue. When you've made a judgment, there is no place to go—there is no room for anything to change.

In establishing boundaries, we want to use our intuition to form opinions, and we want to stop short of being judgmental. If, for example, we meet someone new and have a negative feeling about them, we don't want to ignore that feeling. That intuitive insight could be our inner guidance telling us to take care of ourselves. But how do we ensure that we're not just being judgmental? First, examine the quality and the nature of the insight. Intuition usually happens in an instant, and often has a physical component, such as a flutter or clenching in our stomachs, cold or sweaty palms, lightheadedness, anxiety, or exhaustion.

Intuitive feelings can be difficult to put into words. If asked to explain your feelings, you might find yourself saying something like, "I don't know what it is, but something just doesn't feel (or look, or sound, or seem) right." You may be unable to clearly articulate exactly what feels "off" or dangerous about the situation. You might try and translate the intuitive feeling into what you think might be going on such as, "I don't feel like I can trust that person," or "It feels like they want something from me," or "I just feel like I am supposed to keep my distance." These are not judgmental statements. They are opinions about how being around this person makes you feel. (Of course, you might also have strong positive intuitive feelings about someone and be equally unable to articulate them beyond "I know I don't know her, but there is just something about her I really like.")

If the person who asked you to explain your feelings accepts what you've said, your intuitive feelings and opinions remain open and subject to change. If they argue with the boundary you've just set and ask you to defend your intuition, it's easy to become

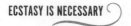

judgmental. How? Well, when our intuition isn't honored—in all its inarticulate truth—we can fall into the trap of trying to justify our intuition by making up reasons (i.e., judgments) that we hope will convince our interrogator to honor our boundary.

EXERCISE: SETTING BOUNDARIES

In your notebook, recall a past incident in which you instinctively knew you should set a boundary, but:

- you let someone talk you out of it, or

- you talked yourself out of it because you thought you were being judgmental, or

- you talked yourself out of it because you had no "proof."

If you could replay this scenario, how would you handle the situation differently today?

Intuitive Empaths and Boundaries

Very intuitive people—sometimes referred to as intuitive empaths, a term coined by Dr. Judith Orloff and explored in depth in her exceptionally popular book *Emotional Freedom*—often require stronger boundaries. We are all intuitive empaths to some extent. Dr. Orloff points to studies of "mirror neurons" which show that brain cells light up not just when your own finger is pricked with a needle, but also when you see someone else's finger being pricked. We actually do feel each other's pain. This is the biological under-pinning of compassion.

Intuitive empaths, moreover, are uber-sensitive and tend to absorb the energy around them. As Dr. Orloff, an empath herself, puts it, "We're super-responders. Our sensory experience of re-lationship is the equivalent of feeling objects with fifty fingers instead of five." I am a lifelong intuitive empath and exhibit all the classic symptoms: I don't like being in crowds, especially cha-otic loud crowds. I avoid parties. I don't socialize very often and when I do I prefer one-on-one dinners or small gatherings. I enjoy being alone. I have become physically ill upon entering buildings, such as a prisons or quarantine camps, where people have been traumatized. I suffer physical symptoms when I'm around people who drain my energy.

I cannot even conceive of living in a group house. When I first moved to New York, I rented a miserable tiny studio that I could afford on my own rather than have to live with a roommate.

Like many intuitive empaths, I have found it challenging to be in intimate relationships. Where many people want to get as close to someone as they can, I need to keep some distance or I will feel smothered and overwhelmed. It was not until well into my 40s that I agreed to live with a romantic partner. Although I was frequently in a relationship, I always needed to keep my own apartment—a room of my own—to escape to for quiet time. I still have that room of my own; this time it is in the apartment my partner and I share. I often work and relax in that room with the door closed, and my partner respects that boundary.

If you are an intuitive empath—and even if you are not—try this exercise to discover the boundaries you might want to set around space and time. This does not just apply to romantic rela-tionships. Friends who wish to travel together or share an apart-ment would do well to examine their needs around space and time before agreeing to share space. You can do this same exercise for a variety of close relationships.

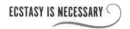

Exercise: Sharing Time and Space

Answer the following questions in your notebook:

Time: Even if you live together, the amount of time you actually spend together can be negotiable. Occasional weekend trips or vacations apart might be soothing and regenerative. Or, you may be able to satisfy your need for alone time by simply arranging to do different activities in different rooms. **How much time do you wish to spend together?**

Activities: For example, some people find showering or bathing together a romantic experience. Others cherish their bathroom time as alone time and do not want company. Ask yourself a similar question about mundane tasks as well. Perhaps you really like to go grocery shopping by yourself. Or maybe you really appreciate companionship when you visit the doctor or dentist. **What kinds of things would you enjoy doing together? What kinds of things would you prefer to do alone?**

Sharing space: Some people need an entire house—or a wing of a house—to themselves. Others need a room or an office. A private closet will satisfy this need for others. **How much private space do you need?**

Traveling: Although I am an adventurous traveler and love visiting friends, I cannot sleep in any room where I cannot close the door. I have been known to hang a sheet or set up a makeshift screen to energetically seal off my room. If I'm sharing a hotel room, I need occasional alone time there. **What are your needs regarding space, time, and activities when you travel?**

Whether you are an intuitive empath or not, your intuition will play a key role in how and where you set your boundaries in relationships. Your intuition is not an excuse that allows you to escape responsibility for your actions and your decisions. But neither is your intuition something that either you or someone else should dismiss as less important or less valid than any other reason for setting a boundary.

Radical Acceptance

It's natural for us to want our lovers and partners to like and want the same things we do. But, obviously, that's not always possible—or even desirable. It's often when we don't like what our partner wants and it becomes necessary to co-create another option, that we step into the Totality of Possibilities.

Radical Acceptance is the art of accepting things exactly the way they are with no expectation that they will change. You make a decision to accept *what* is exactly the *way* it is. Instead of arguing about it, pathologizing it, or trying to change it, you simply accept it. In the acceptance of what is without the expectation of change, countless opportunities appear. The practice of Radical Acceptance can work wonders when we want a loved one to appreciate something that we love, or when we want to communicate with a loved one when we don't like something they love.

My friend, performance artist Annie Sprinkle, is the high priestess of spontaneous and enthusiastic Radical Acceptance. I have learned the practice from her. Annie and I met and began working together in the late 1980s as she was transitioning out of her career as a prostitute and porn actress and into her new career as an AIDS activist and performance artist. We not only became the best of friends, but also partners in art. I was at varying times the producer, manager, production manager, or director of Annie's performance art works for more than ten years. In 2004, Annie and her partner, artist Elizabeth Stevens, began a seven-year series

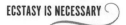

of performance art weddings. Having worked with sex for so many years, Annie now wanted to explore the nature of love—not only love for her partner, but also for humanity, the earth, and for life itself.

I live in New York City, the city Annie and Beth chose for their first wedding. It was an extremely ambitious undertaking, with outrageous costumes, an impressive physical production, and artists flying in from all over the world to participate. Annie wanted me to be the production manager/wedding planner for the event, as well as participate as a performer. I was deeply conflicted about participating. I couldn't imagine not working with Annie on such an important performance event. Yet, there was an enormous stumbling block: I absolutely loathe weddings. Not only do I despise wedding ceremonies, I simply do not believe in the institution of marriage. I see marriage as a violation of the separation of church and state. My antipathy for all things marriage-related is nothing new. As the gay rights movement exploded on the scene in the 1970s, I was idealistically hopeful that the gay community would create a new paradigm that would eventually replace marriage as the prototype for relationships. (What can I say? We all have our starry-eyed, youthful dreams.)

My stomach was in knots as I called Annie. What was I going to tell her? When I finally worked up the courage to make the call, I was in tears. I told her of my horrible dilemma. I wanted to be there for her but I couldn't bear the thought of having to participate in a wedding. Annie, bless her, did not miss a beat. "Let's use this!" she exclaimed. "We'll make art out of it! When the person marrying us asks 'Does anyone object to the union of these two people?' you'll do your performance piece. You'll express all the feelings and opinions you have about marriage. It will be fantastic!"

This is the practice of Radical Acceptance. Annie did not try to change my mind about marriage. She did not tell me that this wedding would be different. She did not try to heal whatever early childhood wounds led to this aversion—she simply accepted it. And that changed everything. Instead of an argument or a weepy fight, Annie and I spent the next 30 minutes outlining my anti-marriage performance piece "Why Marriage Should Be Abolished," which, by the way, was such a huge hit at the wedding that Annie and Beth had other artists perform the piece at several of their subsequent art weddings.

Radical Acceptance is the art of accepting each other's boundaries as they are without needing or expecting them to change. As we all know, the only constant in life is change, so boundaries do stretch and change. But all boundaries need to be accepted and respected in the *present moment*. The more you argue with someone about whether their boundary is reasonable, fair, sensible, or just, the more solid the boundary will become. The more a boundary is respected, the safer a person feels and the more likely it is that the boundary will become more flexible as time passes and conditions shift.

Remember the Resilient Edge of Resistance? What you resist will persist. If you push too hard, whatever you are pushing against will push back—even harder. By ceasing to push against what is not wanted, the pressure is relieved. The situation begins to soften and to change, if only a little.

Use this handy guide when confronted with situations that require Radical Acceptance.

Practicing Radical Acceptance

1. *Accept what is as it is.* E.g., "I know you really don't like or trust my mother. Christmas is coming and she expects us to be there for the holidays."

2. *Look for ways that the situation can work without asking for what is to change.* E.g., "Even though this is true how can we make the holidays a happy time for us?"

3. *Think outside the box.* Brainstorm. Look for possible solutions neither of you has thought of before. E.g., "We could spend Christmas apart. I'll go to my family and you go to yours." Or "We can spend it with your family this year, but we'll stay in a hotel, not in your mother's house. I can certainly make it through one dinner. I like your brother. I can talk with him. Plus, we could arrive late and leave early." Or "We can spend Christmas at home with friends, and visit neither family." Or "Let's not celebrate Christmas with family this year. Let's go to Aruba—just the two of us!"

Radical Acceptance goes beyond simply accepting that things are the way they are. Radical Acceptance practiced at its highest level—and this is the radical part—means enthusiastically embracing the way things are as an opportunity for finding infinitely more creative and ecstatic possibilities.

Often, "finding a compromise" means that no one is happy with the result, but agrees they can live with it. This sort of conditional acceptance virtually eliminates an avenue for a potentially ecstatic experience. There is no energy generated. At best, the compromise will stop the situation from draining your energy. Moreover, when we make compromise after compromise after compromise, there is simply not enough energy being generated in the relationship, the job, or the situation to fuel ecstasy.

Remember the phrase "When life hands you lemons make lemonade?" When presented with lemons, many of us try to make pomegranate juice, or iced tea—flavored with a hint of lemon. It simply doesn't work. Radical Acceptance means creating the most delicious, tongue-tingling lemonade you can, with no pretense that it's anything else.

Radical Acceptance does not mean that you have to agree with someone's boundary or choice. It does not mean that you must ignore your own needs. Radical Acceptance is a practice much like forgiveness, in that you do not practice forgiveness in order to make the other person right. You practice forgiveness to release yourself from the bondage of the past. You forgive in order to become free. Similarly, you practice Radical Acceptance to disengage from a potential or actual tug-of-war. You practice Radical Acceptance to become benignly detached.

Radical Acceptance does not mean settling for something that's not acceptable to you. When you practice Radical Acceptance you get to choose from a Totality of Possibilities. Among those possibilities is walking away, saying no, or choosing not to participate. If Annie had needed only people who were 100 percent in support of marriage at her wedding, she could have accepted my feelings and the fact that I could not be there. I could also have accepted that I could not be there. We could have made plans to see each other and spend time together before or after the wedding. In more challenging situations, Radical Acceptance can lead to solutions that can dramatically alter the fabric of a relationship, or even end it. Even—and perhaps especially—in these cases, you step into a completely new chapter in your Totality of Possibilities.

Radical Acceptance works in even the most sensitive situations. In my coaching practice I often work with men and couples who are coping with premature ejaculation and erectile dysfunction. Often by the time they find me, they are sad and frustrated.

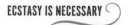

The men feel broken, the women blame themselves. When we approach the problem with Radical Acceptance we acknowledge that these conditions happen sometimes. We give the condition permission to exist and ask what opportunities it may present. There are thousands of ways to be sexual. Intercourse with an erect penis which can ejaculate at just the right moment is only one of them. There are plenty of ways for both partners to show each other love and intimacy and give each other orgasms while premature ejaculation and erectile dysfunction are part of the equation. I suggest these couples try oral sex, sex toys, breathwork, sensual massage, and an infinite variety of exquisite erotic massage techniques. When we are done the couple has a dozen or more new erotic scenarios that excite them. Usually, this alone will lower the instances of premature ejaculation and erectile dysfunction, but in cases where the problem has a physical cause and is not so easily remedied, the couple can still enjoy a terrific sex life.

Radical Acceptance is an invitation to greater creativity and personal growth. Many people find the experience of Radical Acceptance so liberating and exhilarating that the practice alone becomes an ecstatic experience.

EXERCISE: RETROACTIVE RADICAL ACCEPTANCE

In your notebook, describe a situation in your past that could have benefited from the practice of Radical Acceptance. Describe how you might have accepted what was exactly the way it was, and list at least three creative possibilities that might have resulted.

Sexual Preference and Gender Identity

Our boundaries are part of our identity. They tell us who we are and who we aren't, who and what we are or aren't attracted to.

Nowhere is this more clear or obvious than in the areas of gender identity and sexual preference.

Gender identity and sexual preference are often mistakenly lumped together in one category. They are actually completely different. Your gender identity answers the question "Who am I?" Your sexual preference answers the question "Who am I attracted to?" Both gender identity and sexual preference were once seen as fixed binaries. The only two choices for a gender identity were male and female, and the only acceptable choice for a sexual preference was someone of the "opposite" gender. If you weren't perfectly gendered—meaning you did not fit neatly and obviously into either the male or female category—*and* have the correct sexual preference, your boundaries around your gender identity and sexual preference weren't considered worthy of being honored. You could be arrested in a gay bar, beaten up on the street, or forced into programs designed to change your sexual preference or gender identity.

Until relatively recently, even professionals who worked with differently gendered people could not fully comprehend the difference between gender identity and sexual preference. For example, transgender people once faced a huge hurdle in being approved for genital reassignment surgery if their sexual preferences did not line up with their gender identity. In the mid-1980s, my partner, Kate, was refused genital reassignment surgery by several surgeons because none of them could conceive of the possibility of a lesbian transsexual.

Luckily, human rights and social norms have taken a few steps forward in recent decades, at least in many areas of the world. We are gradually weaning ourselves away from binary thinking in more and more areas of life, including gender identity and sexual preference. More and more of us are able to think of gender and sexual preference as a rainbow spectrum along which everyone can find the particular shade of color that looks best on them. It is no longer as simple as man or woman, homosexual or heterosexual.

Many people will shift their gender in some significant way over the course of their lifetime. This does not mean that everyone is transgendered or transsexual. A change of gender can be as simple and obvious as a woman taking on a job that has traditionally been done by men—or a man climbing down the corporate ladder to become a stay-at-home dad. Many people's sexual preferences will also change in some significant way. A heterosexual woman might suddenly find herself attracted to a female friend. A man might realize that he's always been bisexual. Many people come to realize that the gender of their partner has little to do with their attraction to that partner.

Sexual preference does not just refer to who we are attracted to, but also to the kind of erotic activities we are attracted to. I have friends and clients whose sexual tastes have changed from a fondness for BDSM to a passion for Tantra, and vice versa. A few have gone a step further and are combining BDSM and Tantra. In both cases, boundaries have had to change as sexual preferences changed.

Each of us has the right to change our gender identity or sexual preference as many times over the course of our lifetime as we like. Each time we make a new choice we need to set new boundaries. For example, someone going through a gender change will likely want to be called by a new name. A heterosexual woman who becomes a lesbian will ask men to respect the fact that she is not going to have sex with them. It is crucial but not always easy to respect people's boundaries as their identities and preferences shift and grow—as the following story illustrates.

After 30 years of marriage, Dean, in his late 50s, finally made the decision that he wanted to live the rest of his life as a woman. This was not a bizarre symptom of a late midlife crisis, but rather a profound realization arrived at after 50 years of trying to deny his femininity. Dean's wife, Betsy, loved Dean deeply, but as you can imagine, was seriously confused. Betsy's identity and sexual preferences were now completely thrown into question. If she stayed with Dean (now calling herself Deana) was she still a wife? Was she a lesbian? Would she be attracted to Deana when the feminizing power of the female hormones Deana was taking became more apparent? What were Betsy's own needs in this process? And what were her boundaries?

Betsy went into therapy, prayed, and looked at the issue from as many sides as she possibly could. In the end, she found the practice of Radical Acceptance the most helpful. Her husband was becoming her wife. Who was to say that might not be a fun thing? She realized that although this process was enormously challenging, she was finding out things about herself and about Deana that she had never discovered before. She was also learning how to set firm yet flexible boundaries to make the process easier to manage emotionally.

What Betsy appreciated most was the opportunity to embrace the values of creativity, flexibility, and spontaneity that she had always cherished intellectually, but never really felt she had embodied. Deana and Betsy had long shared a love of adventure, and this new chapter in their lives certainly met that value. Plus, the completely new experience of having a live-in best girlfriend was a delight in itself. All in all, Betsy discovered her new Totality of Possibilities was definitely more of an energy gain than an energy drain. Betsy and Deana's relationship developed a decidedly ecstatic new dimension that was rapidly expanding.

The ecstatic realm is not available to us if we limit our gender expression or sexual preferences to something others find easily acceptable. It may feel like we are being considerate or respectful to others when we pretend to be someone we aren't, but it does not work for long, and denies us the ecstatic possibilities of our authenticity.

The path to ecstasy is peppered with paradoxes. Gender and sexual preference present us with this one: Although both ecstatic experiences and ecstatic relationships are characterized by a boundlessness and expansiveness, one needs to be very clear about one's boundaries in order to be able to dance in the ecstasy.

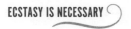

EXERCISE: GENDER AND SEX

In your notebook, write down three ways in which your gender expression has shifted in the past ten years. (Hint: Aging is a shift in gender all by itself.)

Write down three (or more) ways in which your sexual preferences have changed. (Reminder: Sexual preference does not only refer to who we are attracted to, but also to the kind of erotic activities we are attracted to.)

Others-in-Law

From both spiritual and scientific perspectives, we know that we are all connected, all part of a great whole. Any individual action taken by one person affects every other part of the whole, however lightly or dramatically. The concept of six degrees of separation (also referred to as the "human web") demonstrates that everyone on earth can be connected to anyone else on earth in six or fewer "friend of a friend" steps.

On a personal level, we are all in relationship with everyone with whom our friends, family, and lovers are in relationship even if we seldom see them. Whether it's their mother, sister, brother, cousin, boss, child, or—in the case of people in non-monogamous relationships—other lovers. Even if you have never met your boyfriend's boss, you know you are in relationship with his boss when your boyfriend calls and once again cancels a weekend trip with you because she has yet another emergency she expects your boyfriend to handle. I call the significant others in our beloveds' lives our others-in-law. As anyone with problematical in-laws can attest, nothing can drain the ecstasy out of a relationship as fast as a disagreement over the others-in-law.

In the next chapter, we'll look at the importance of community or tribe as a source of support in building sexual courage. When we add new and more people to the mix, we also weave a web that

128

includes all their relations—we connect with even more others-in-law. Learning how to form your own boundaries and respect those of your others-in-law is key to establishing the sustainable erotic, ecstatic relationships that form the foundation of ecstatic experiences.

People will experience some degree of one of three relationship dynamics: attraction, repulsion, and neutrality. In purely scientific terms, this is true for any two objects.

In pharmacology, for example, a drug that can combine with a cell's receptor to produce some physiologic reaction is called an agonist. A drug that blocks or reverses the effect of the agonist is an antagonist. Often, the same substance can be either an agonist or an antagonist, depending on the dose. The hormone pregnenolone, for example, is a sedative at low doses. At high doses, it causes agitation and a racing heartbeat.

Similarly, someone you seldom see and hardly know may be perfectly pleasant in small doses. However, if they become your other-in-law and you are expected to interact with them on a regular basis, they may become a stress-producing antagonist.

How do we establish appropriate boundaries with less-than-appealing others-in-law without damaging our primary relationship? What is an appropriate relationship with any other-in-law?

This is an area fraught with expectations. We may expect that everyone who loves us will love—or at least like—each other. We may expect that when we form a relationship with someone that they will seamlessly flow into our extended network of others. We may expect that everyone will at least pretend to like each other even if they don't. In the best of all possible worlds, all of this happens. Often it doesn't.

This discussion is not meant to predict, affirm, or presuppose that you won't find yourself enveloped into a supportive and loving new family or constellation of friends. But when you do not get along with one or more of your others-in-law, you often feel the same way you do when you find yourself in a less-than-fulfilling sexual relationship, i.e., that you are somehow wrong, at fault, broken, different, and/or alone in your feelings.

However, as any support group for members of dysfunctional stepfamilies will tell you, this problem is exceedingly common.

Practicing Radical Acceptance can be challenging when dealing with others-in-law, but it's certainly possible, as my friend Ellie's story proves. Ellie disliked her daughter Sara's new boyfriend, Ted, instantly. As she described it, "I hated him—just hated him." Ted was very upset that Ellie didn't like him. He tried everything to make a good impression on her. This in fact, was the problem. He was trying far too hard. Ellie never had an opportunity to see Ted's true self. Sara tried to point this out to Ted. She suggested he stop working so hard and just be himself. Ted could not seem to do this, so nothing changed. Ted remained upset; Ellie didn't want to have anything to do with him. It was Sara who first began to practice Radical Acceptance. She did not try to convince Ellie that Ted was a wonderful guy. After her initial suggestion to Ted that he just be himself, she didn't try to persuade him to do anything differently. She told each of them "I love Ted and I love my mom. How you two feel about each other will not change my love for either of you."

And then Sara did nothing but show both her boyfriend and her mom that she loved them both deeply. She did not try to persuade Ellie that she was wrong about Ted, nor did she concoct situations to force them to spend time together. She just loved them both and got on with her life. For a while, nothing substantial changed between Ted and Ellie, but with no pressure from Sara, both of them began to relax a bit. They could at least accept each other's presence in Sara's life.

One day Ellie got very sick. She called Sara's house and Ted answered. He told Ellie that Sara was several hours away on business. Did she want him to come over? "No," she said. "I'll be fine. Just tell her I called." When Sara arrived home three hours later Ted greeted her at the door with a packed suitcase. "Your mother called," he said. "She needs you. Get back in the car. Here's your bag. There are enough clothes in it for a few days. Call me if there is anything I can do."

That one gesture changed everything. When Sara got to Ellie's house and told her what had happened, Ellie saw her first glimpse of who Ted was, rather than who he was trying to be. Beginning with that moment, their relationship grew and deepened. Today they genuinely love each other.

In difficult other-in-law situations, Radical Acceptance, respect for each other's boundaries, plus a bit of patience, can work wonders. When you allow the winds of change to dance between you, the universe can work miracles. But, you may ask, how does one cope in the meantime?

If you, like Sara, are positioned between two others-in-law who do not get along, ask yourself, how important is it for me that these two people get along? Will they be seeing each other on a regular basis? If the warring parties are your fiancé and your teenage daughter, very different considerations are in play than if the disagreement is between your fiancé and a friend who lives a thousand miles away. You could affirm, "My mother's and my fiancé's opinion of each other has nothing to do with me. I love them; they love me. We are safe." Above all, do not force, cajole, manipulate, or nag people into being in relationship with one another. Any sort of coercion is virtually certain to create resentment and hostility.

If you, like Ted, are the person who is disliked by an other-in-law, take a deep breath. Try the following affirmation, "Other people's opinions of me are none of my business. I am surrounded by love. I am safe." Increase the time you spend with people who adore you. Ask them to tell you why they love you. Set an appropriate boundary with the other-in-law who dislikes you.

If you, like Ellie, are in the position of being the one who dislikes an other-in-law, it is helpful to remember that when your intuition tells you to stay away from someone you are most likely picking up on their insecurities, their weaknesses, and their fears. Try to bring empathy to the situation. You might start by affirming, "My daughter's boyfriends are none of my business. My daughter is safe and so am I." After a while, you might be able to silently greet your other-in-law with "Namaste" whenever you think of them. The meaning of Namaste can range from "I respect the spirit in you," to "The Divine in me recognizes the Divine in you." Practice thinking increasingly positive thoughts about your other-in-law, and be open to change.

One of the most stressful situations for everyone involved is when the clashing others-in-law are a stepparent and a minor child. My friend Ingrid's story—which played out over 30 years—illustrates how Radical Acceptance and strong boundaries can bring healing to even the most extreme other-in-law situations.

My friend Ingrid was born in Sweden. She met and fell in love with Ian, a professor at a Midwestern college, when she came to the United States to study. When they met, Ian was living with his 12-year-old son Michael, who had moved in with him less than a year before. Ian and his wife, Michael's mother, had divorced when Michael was four. Prior to living with Ian, Michael had lived in another state with his mom and an abusive stepfather. Michael's mother had sent him to live with his father—thrown him out of the house, really—when she could no longer control him. Michael suffered from oppositional defiant disorder. ODD is characterized by persistent patterns of tantrums, arguing, and angry, disruptive behaviors toward parents and other authority figures.

Ingrid married Ian when Michael was 13. Living together was problematical from the start. Michael hated all mother figures and objected to everything Ingrid said and did. If Ingrid mentioned that rain was expected that day, Michael would start an angry fight about how she didn't know what she was talking about and how stupid she was. When he wasn't openly berating and humiliating her, he was attempting to control the family with power games and one-upmanship.

Ian felt guilty that he had not been there for his son for most of his life and felt partially responsible for Michael's abuse, his ODD, and his behavior. Although Ian loved Ingrid deeply he couldn't help being more concerned about Michael's problems than Ingrid's. Despite intensive family counseling sessions, nothing much changed. After more than two years of this, Ingrid went back to Sweden for a month, just to have a break and to consider her situation.

When she returned to the U.S. they all went back into counseling, but still nothing changed. By now Michael was 16 and things were at a breaking point. Although he was a genius—at age 15 he had a computer programming job and was earning an excellent salary—he had been thrown out of several schools and his behavior toward Ingrid was still uncontrollably hostile.

Ingrid and Ian had hoped that they could make their living situation tolerable until Michael went away to college, but that was still two years away. Having tried everything she and several therapists could think of, Ingrid decided she could not live in this situation any longer. She simply could not put up with being humiliated every single day. Yet, she loved Ian and did not want a divorce.

There was only one solution Ingrid could think of. She rented herself an apartment near Ian's university and moved out of Ian's house. This way she and Ian could have time alone together regularly and she only had to see Michael over an occasional meal once or twice a week when she visited Ian.

Ingrid lived in her apartment happily and successfully for two years. Interestingly enough, both Ian and Michael joined Ingrid in their own version of Radical Acceptance—the new housing situation worked well for everyone. Finally, Michael turned 18 and went off to college—a thousand miles away. Ingrid moved back in with Ian.

Michael is now an adult. He lives on the west coast. He and his dad still have a close relationship. Ingrid made one more attempt to establish a relationship with Michael but it did not work. Michael comes to visit for a few days a couple of times each year. Following the template that Ingrid created when Michael was 16, Ingrid leaves the house when Michael comes to visit. She travels to places she likes, or she goes to visit friends. She loves her alone time and considers it a welcome vacation.

Ian continues to practice Radical Acceptance. He wishes things could be different, but he knows they cannot. Ian's emotional journey began in angst and anguish, moved through disappointment, and has arrived at a sort of wistfulness. He can rest easily here. There is no longer a huge energy drain on his spirit and on his relationships with Michael and Ingrid. The lack of strain has actually become something of an energy gain as peace has replaced anguish.

Ian and Ingrid went through long periods when they both felt like failures as parents and partners. They had no support group, no tribe, and no close family. They knew no one else who was going through anything similar. They came to Radical Acceptance because it was that or give up on their relationship. We often choose to break up when our boundaries clash. It's a common, more familiar choice. Radical Acceptance requires not only creativity, but courage, a subject I'll discuss in the next chapter. It was Radical Acceptance that allowed Ingrid and Ian to find a solution that not only saved their marriage, but allowed it to thrive, as it does, some 30 years later.

Exercise: Boundaries and Radical Acceptance

Part One: Name a situation in your life that requires you to set a boundary. Perhaps you have been hesitant to set this limit, or wishy-washy about its enforcement. In your notebook, write down this boundary exactly as you would like it to be. Do not judge yourself or your boundary. This is not the time to ask whether your boundary is reasonable, appropriate, or justified. Nor will you worry about who may be upset with it. Just state the boundary.

Now, apply Radical Acceptance. Breathe. Accept your boundary exactly the way it is. Imagine others receiving your boundary with Radical Acceptance. Imagine engaging in a creative conversation where your boundary becomes the starting point for an ecstatic solution.

Write down three creative possibilities that might result from enthusiastic acceptance of this boundary.

Part Two: Name a situation in your life that requires you to accept someone else's boundary. In your notebook, write down their boundary as they have stated it to you. (Don't worry about being exact; just come as close as you can.) Perhaps you've been arguing with them about it, or trying to engineer some circumstance in which you hope they'll realize that they are wrong about this boundary. Try not to be judgmental with yourself or with them. This is not the time to ask whether their boundary is reasonable, appropriate, or justified. Just state the boundary.

Now, apply Radical Acceptance. Breathe. Accept their boundary exactly the way it is. Allow it to just be. Imagine engaging in a creative conversation where their boundary becomes the starting point for an ecstatic solution. Practice detachment.

Write down three creative possibilities that might result from enthusiastic acceptance of this boundary.

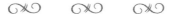

Now that you have a foundation of safety and have established some boundaries, it's time to think about taking an erotic risk. Take a big breath and let's go.

CHAPTER 5

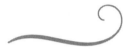

Erotic Risk-taking: Playing with Fire

In Chapter 3 we learned that peak sexual experiences are the result of just the right combination of safety and risk. In this chapter you'll learn how to build or expand your sexual courage for the purpose of taking an erotic risk. You won't need to muster the kind of bravery it takes to step onto a battlefield. Under most battle conditions, feelings of duty or conscription combine with danger and fear to produce the adrenaline necessary to transmute fear into action. Sexual courage is quite different. When you take an erotic risk, you actually have a *strong desire* for the experience you're afraid of. This desire is commonly experienced as a physical longing that pulls your body toward the experience about which your mind may be hesitant. As you will come to see, desire is not only your motivating force, but also your safety belt when you want to take a new erotic risk.

Think of your erotic courage as a muscle. In order to become strong enough to hike the most ecstatic trails, you have to build up this muscle. You'll also need to stretch that same muscle, so it will have the flexibility and stamina to go the distance. Erotic courage is simply the willingness to expand and grow stronger. It's the readiness and the enthusiasm to step further into your Totality of Possibilities—and one step closer to your Something More.

Building courage and erotic self-esteem go hand in hand. Like yin and yang, one constantly flows into and around the other. When we build up our courage, our self-esteem increases; when we build our self-esteem, we exhibit more courage. So, in what circumstances do we think we need to muster courage and/or self-esteem? How about when . . .

. . . we think we aren't enough?
. . . something we want to try has previously failed?
. . . we're trying something new and different?
. . . we're afraid of losing what we have?
. . . we're afraid of being embarrassed or ashamed?

We do not build erotic courage for the purpose of going into battle against some inner or outer force that must be conquered before we can find ecstasy.

Erotically speaking, it is wasteful and counterproductive to use our energy fighting against our own thoughts and feelings, or against the opinions of others. Our energy is far better spent focusing on a pleasurable or ecstatic intention.

Nor do you have to muster the courage to do something huge, outrageous, or uncharacteristically bold. (Although if that is exactly what you *want* to do, I promise I'll give you a step-by-step plan for doing it.) *You need just enough courage to embrace your own authenticity*—however meek or wild that might be.

Here are a few ways to build erotic courage and stretch and strengthen your risk-taking muscles.

Think Outside the Box

One of the first steps in building sexual courage is learning to do things differently, think outside of the box—break some molds. Often we stifle our creative thoughts before we even begin to think them. A stern, internal judge says, "Don't even go there. What would people think?"

My friend Marilyn is a good example of someone who has learned the magic of creative thinking. Marilyn loves building, fixing, and tinkering. She is absolutely ecstatic when she can find a few free hours to spend in her shop in the basement of her house, inventing clever repairs or creating beautiful handcrafted clocks. Marilyn would like to sell her house and move into a condominium. She spent weekend after weekend searching for a new home. She was disappointed in each one because they all lacked a proper space for her shop. I accompanied Marilyn on one of her condo shopping adventures and indeed, there was no typical shop space—i.e., a space tucked away in a basement or a back room—in any of the condos we looked at.

What these condos did all have were living rooms and dining rooms that I knew Marilyn would seldom use. She's not a big socializer and when she does have guests over they will be far more likely to hang out in the kitchen or the den. I suggested she put her shop in either the dining room or the living room. What the heck? It would be her house. Why couldn't she design it any way she liked? Marilyn had never considered that. The real estate agent initially looked horrified, but quickly came around when she saw that this "crazy" thinking might result in a sale. (It's amazing how flexible people become in their opinions when they realize there might be a profit in it.) Marilyn has still not found the right condo, but it's no longer because of a lack of space for her shop. Now when she looks for a condo, she first finds the room for her shop, then she looks at the rest of the space. Thinking outside the box has completely transformed her home-buying experience.

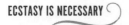

Erotically speaking, thinking outside the box is similarly grati-fying. I worked with a young couple, Christy and Josh, whose sex life had been reduced to what they described as "duty sex" after Christy had a long series of medical procedures that eventually re-sulted in the removal of a particularly stubborn ovarian cyst. This process left both Christy and Josh feeling as though her genitals had become completely medicalized, and therefore de-eroticized. They were having sex because marriage is "supposed" to include sex, and because they feared their relationship might fall apart without it. Needless to say, the duty sex was as—or more—numb-ing than no sex at all. Christy and Josh needed permission to think outside of the box. I suggested they stop having sex for a while or reinvent sex. They chose to reinvent sex. They dropped penis-vagina intercourse from their repertoire and focused instead on erotic massage and role-play. They also stopped trying to have "maintenance" sex of any kind and instead, committed to longer but less frequent sessions of lovemaking. It was a big risk, and both of them were apprehensive—but it worked. They rediscovered their passion in these more creative, playful, and intense sessions. They discovered that two or three hot, exciting sexual experiences a month were more nourishing than a steady diet of mundane sex.

EXERCISE: CHANGE A HABIT

Do you have a food habit? Perhaps you eat the same thing for breakfast or lunch every day. Or maybe you have the same bever-age or snack every day at 4 P.M. Try something new. Have a salad for breakfast—or ice cream! Have eggs for lunch—or a new flavor of coffee or tea at 4 P.M.

Find Inspiration

Often we feel yearnings pulling us toward a new adventure, but we can't imagine what that adventure might be. These soul cravings can feel like a longing for something missing or unknown, but just as frequently, a craving can feel like an itch that just has to be scratched.

My friend Janet loves to bake bread. Over the course of the past winter Janet felt that she had put on too much weight and decided she'd stop baking for a while. The temptation to eat all the yummy things she created was just too great. She put out a call to her friends for suggestions for a substitute hobby, and received numerous ideas, ranging from taking long walks to candle making and embroidery. None of the suggestions felt quite right to Janet. As she put it, none of them seemed to "scratch the same itch" as baking bread. Once she described it that way, it was easy to understand what she was looking for. Almost instantly, someone suggested making sculptures with clay, which, of course, was extremely similar to kneading bread dough. Perfect! Janet had found her new hobby.

You can make the decision to use this same self-loving mindset and process when looking for new erotic inspiration.

Where is your soul itching to take you?

My clients Melissa and Gregory came to me because Gregory was suffering from erectile dysfunction. Happily, both Melissa and Gregory were well onto the path of Radical Acceptance of this situation. They felt comfortable and easy discussing the problem with each other and with me, and neither of them was blaming the other. Melissa and Gregory had always really enjoyed intercourse. It wasn't that they had never explored or enjoyed other sexual activities—they simply loved having intercourse. Gregory's erectile dysfunction was, therefore, a serious blow to their relationship. They were both sad and discouraged. We discussed a wide variety of sexual activities that could bring them both pleasure without intercourse. Melissa was not overly enthused with any of them. I asked her, "What would scratch the same itch as intercourse?" "Frankly," she said, "being penetrated and fucked really hard. Edward has been using his fingers, but it's not the same thing." "Have you considered a dildo?" I asked. There was a pause. "Honestly," she said, "yes, I have. But I thought it would be too humiliating for Gregory." Much to her surprise, Gregory was completely open to the idea. His greatest upset about his condition was that he could not pleasure Melissa in the way he had been able to. I suggested that they could begin with Gregory holding the dildo in his hand, but Gregory was way ahead of me. "Is it possible to strap on one of those things?" he asked. "Indeed it is," I told him. Melissa and Gregory left the session a few minutes early to go shopping at the sex toy store.

Melissa's first notions about the dildo had come to her in a fantasy. She had been masturbating and had slipped into a fantasy of Gregory strapping on a brightly colored dildo. In her fantasy the dildo did not have anything to do with his erectile dysfunction—it was just a hot image that really turned her on.

Our fantasies are potent sources of inspiration and can give us clues about the erotic and ecstatic adventures we'd like to take. Certainly, we cannot live out all our fantasies. Many of our fantasies would be either dangerous or impossible to play out in real life. But fantasy gives us clues to our longings.

If you are wondering how to find inspiration for your next adventure into "Something More," set aside time to daydream.

Whether it's lying on a beach, walking in the woods, masturbation, or meditation, give yourself space to dream and fantasize. Push beyond old familiar fantasies into something new and fresh. Breathe. Use your breath to keep your attention on your intention: creative new erotic and ecstatic scenarios.

142

My colleague and friend Denise Linn asks an especially effective and inspiring question in her past-life regression workshops: "If you knew what you wanted, what would it be?" This question is adaptable to any situation in which you need to access both imagination and deeper knowing.

- If you knew where you were going, where would that be?

- If you knew who you were looking for, who would that be?

- If you knew what erotic risk you wanted to take next, what would that be?

- If you knew who you wanted to take an erotic risk with, who would that be?

- If you knew how you wanted to feel after your next ecstatic experience, what would that feeling be?

Other good sources of inspiration are books and blogs—especially erotic memoirs and story collections. Pornography is a great source of erotic inspiration, if you choose the porn that works for you. I recommend porn made by filmmakers such as Tristan Taormino, Nina Hartley, Candida Royalle, and Erika Lust, who have high standards and an intention to inspire and educate, as well as entertain. You can find quality erotica at independent, feminist, local stores such as Smitten Kitten, Come As You Are, Good For Her, and Early to Bed, just to name a few. All have online catalogs. Be cautious of any porn that portrays people as emotionless sexbots acting out extreme and impossible scenarios.

Another great source of inspiration is other people. There is a lot to be learned from voyeuring. It's perfectly okay to just watch, so long as it's done in a discreet, respectful manner. Many groups actually encourage voyeuring by having specific guidelines for people who just want to watch. Common rules include asking permission, not getting too close, and keeping conversation to a minimum. I'll

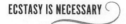

talk more about groups and erotic communities later in this chapter. Whether your passions are sexual, spiritual, or kinky, watching other people play can be a great source of creativity and insight.

Be Willing to Be Uncomfortable

The path to ecstasy is not always comfortable. Nothing great, noble, profound, or ecstatic has ever been achieved by someone who is primarily concerned with staying safely within their comfort zone. The path to peak experience is frequently paved with physical, emotional, and spiritual challenges. As my partner Kate says, "Ships are safe in harbor—but that's not what ships are built for."

Anyone who's ever taken a yoga class or embarked upon an exercise program knows that the process is not always easy or pleasant. In your first class or session, you may have been physically uncomfortable because your muscles were out of shape. You may have been emotionally uncomfortable because you were embarrassed that you weren't up to the rest of the class or others in the gym. You may have been spiritually uncomfortable because while you were still learning the yoga postures you weren't feeling any of the meditative benefits you were expecting. However, as you worked your way through your discomforts, you found strength, pleasure, and a sense of accomplishment and serenity, all of which combined to produce a positive experience. The same thing is true of more extreme ecstatic endeavors.

Allow me to take you back to the ball dance that someone chose as their peak ecstatic experience in Chapter 1. Being pierced with needles and having weights and decorations sewn into the skin is not comfortable for most people. The needles are not intensely painful, but neither are they the ecstatic part of the adventure. Moreover, one's first steps into the dance after the weights have been sewn on are also not painful, but also not entirely comfortable, because the body has not yet produced sufficient endorphins. But when the drums are pounding and your dance is in full flight, you have not only completely transcended discomfort; you have soared into an ecstatic trance.

Emotional uneasiness is also a part of the process when we step out of our comfort zone into our as-yet-unknown Something More. A new erotic or ecstatic activity opens us to a new level of intimacy with ourselves, and with others. Being exposed to any new levels of intensity can be scary. Just like in the gym or in yoga class, your first attempts may be stiff and awkward. However, if you take a deeper breath and allow yourself to fall further into the posture or exercise, it first becomes less painful, then less uncomfortable, and finally, perfect.

Riding the ever-shifting Resilient Edges of Resistance of our bodies and our emotions necessitates being uncomfortable for a moment or two. After all, it's not until we notice that we are uncomfortable that we shift our position. Think about it. Imagine sitting cross-legged on the floor, about to meditate. You are completely comfortable and feel like you could sit like this forever. However, after a few minutes, one of your legs begins to hurt. Eventually you need to switch your position somewhat or your leg will go numb. You shift in order to meet this new resilient edge. In this way, you make yourself comfortable enough to stay in the present moment.

Have you ever held hands with a beloved until both your hands were so sweaty and cramped that what had started as a warm, intimate connection had become a painful and unpleasant experience? You didn't break up or get angry. You simply changed position—perhaps you put your arms around each other instead—so that your intimate connection could continue.

When we experience an initial feeling of discomfort shortly into the process of trying something new or taking some new risk—especially an erotic or ecstatic risk—it helps to use the affirmation "I make no judgments, no comparisons, and I release my need to understand." The present moment is our point of power. When we can sit with our physical or emotional discomfort, breathe into it and embrace it with Radical Acceptance, it will begin to shift. We will be guided into the change we need to make in order to allow us to continue on our ecstatic journey.

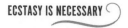
Surrender

Surrender—even to a higher power—is not something our culture encourages. Surrender is giving up the need to control. We cross over from our well-defined roles and worlds into the realm of the gods, where everything is possible and nothing is explained. This is scary stuff. The word surrender—having been commandeered by governments and military forces—conjures up images of defeat rather than release. Nevertheless, in order to reach your ecstatic bliss, your Something More, your Totality of Possibilities, your highest self—you must surrender.

Surrender—either to a person or a force—is not the same act as submission. To ecstatic explorers, surrender doesn't mean voluntarily submitting to unpleasant experiences. Surrender is not at all the same as "grin and bear it." Surrender is not giving up or giving in. Surrender is a conscious choice.

Some people find it much easier to surrender when that surrender is explicit and consensual, such as in S/M, bondage, and dominant/submissive role-playing. Others find that sort of explicit surrender brings up all their control issues. Everyone's path to and method of surrender is unique and valid.

I sometimes explain surrender to my workshop participants in the same way as I describe releasing expectations before a breath and energy orgasm. I find that the best attitude is something along the lines of "Oh, what the fuck? I've already invested a couple of hours in this workshop. I may as well breathe and see what happens."

Breathe. Allow a softness to permeate your being. Let go.

> You will have no enemies once you decide to surrender. Surrender means
> not giving in to another but giving in to love.
>
> — DEEPAK CHOPRA

I consistently ask the participants in my workshops to take erotic and ecstatic risks. Therefore, I think it's only fair that I maintain a regular risk-taking routine of my own. I love learning new things, so my erotic risks frequently involve acquiring a new skill, as well as embracing a new experience. Some months after my erotic risk in the fMRI machine, I felt the need for a new adventure.

Not long after I'd stated my intention to find something new to explore, I attended a conference where I witnessed a presentation of a skill-based activity I had never tried before. I was enthralled—and terrified. I decided to sign up for a weekend workshop, scheduled six months later, that would teach me how to pursue this activity on a professional level. I kept a journal of my entire process—from my decision to take this risk through the workshop itself—with all its emotional ups and downs and ups again. I then reduced my journal to an outline in order to examine the steps I had followed: deciding to take the risk, navigating my way through the risk, and finally, experiencing the ecstatic reward from having taken the risk.

I offer this outline of my process as a prototype for erotic risk-taking. Obviously, different erotic risks require different specifics and this model may not be entirely applicable to all erotic or ecstatic situations. However, it is highly adaptable for different circumstances and will provide you with a solid model for an initial approach.

Ecstatic Risk-taking in Ten Simple Steps

Erotic risk-taking is not an all-or-nothing process. It's a series of manageable steps that take you from initial interest to ecstatic fulfillment at a pace that is comfortable.

1. Find your turn-on.

The first step in taking an erotic or ecstatic risk is finding something about the risk that excites you. At the erotic conference I attended, an old friend of mine, Fakir Musafar, was presenting several workshops. In the world of BDSM and body modification,

Fakir is a legend. He is an artist, shaman, and a master piercer. Fakir has played a hugely significant role in the modern revival of body modification, including piercing, branding, and body sculpting. He is a co-developer of the modern body-piercing techniques in general use today. The intentions behind all of Fakir's work are personal expression, spiritual exploration, rites of passage, and healing.

Annie Sprinkle had introduced me to Fakir some 20 years earlier when she and I were exploring Tantra and other forms of sacred sexuality. Fakir and I would regularly get lost in long conversations about the sacred dimensions he had found in the extended, expanded ecstatic states of intense endurance rituals, such as re-enactments of the Native American sundance ritual, Indian kavadi dances, ball dancing, hook pulls, and hook suspensions. At the time, I was nowhere near ready to try any of these, but I was deeply attracted to his description of the transcendental states that seemed so similar to my experiences with Tantric sex.

Over the years, I saw Fakir less frequently, as he lives in California and I live in New York. But my attraction to the practices we had talked about grew stronger. Initially, I voyeured and got high off the energy of the other participants. Slowly, step-by-step, I experimented with my own versions of some of his work. When I felt inclined to take a risk and try something new, I did just that. Along the way, I received numerous piercings and several tattoos. I even learned how to do a little bit of basic body piercing.

The one thing I never tried—and up to this point had never even witnessed—was branding. Like lots of people, I thought of branding as something you did to cows with a heavy, metal hot poker. This seemed scary and not at all erotic to me. However, if anyone could practice branding as a Zen art form, it was Fakir. It just so happened that he was teaching a branding workshop at the erotic conference we were attending. Curious as I was, I sat at the back of the room just in case it was all too much for me. Fakir began by debunking the many myths about branding, including the myth about the red-hot iron poker. He showed us the tiny, ever-so-thin pieces of metal, which he could bend into all sorts of delicate patterns. Fakir placed these bits of metal into a vise grip and heated them with a propane torch till they were glowing red hot—approximately 2,400 degrees Fahrenheit. At this temperature these tiny pieces of metal would kill nerve endings on contact, which meant that the branding process was less painful than one might think. Learning this single fact reduced my fear factor immeasurably.

I'd stumbled upon branding as something completely new, different, and frightening—only to find that I was attracted to branding because it was similar to something I already love: fire. Fire is a huge sensual and sexual turn-on for me. I regularly use fire as a key element in my workshops and rituals. (I have a degree in fire eating and fireplay from the Coney Island Sideshow School.) In some of my workshops I even combine fire with massage. I put a little rubbing alcohol on my hand, light the alcohol on fire, and then place my flaming hand on the body on my massage table. The recipient experiences this hot touch as similar to a hot stone massage. It feels wonderfully relaxing to the receiver and I get a chance to play with fire, so it's a turn-on for both of us.

So, the more I learned about the process of branding—and the more frequently Fakir fired up the propane torch—the less afraid and more attracted I was. It was still risky, but oh-so-alluring. I found myself standing up and moving nearer to the table so that I could see everything more closely. As I watched Fakir bend, trim, and shape the little bits of metal that would be used to brand a volunteer's chosen design on her arm, I was captivated by the craft involved. By the time Fakir was actually creating the brand on his eager volunteer's arm, I was so close I was hovering over the table.

It's this emotional/physical pull toward something or some-one that tells me I am turned on. If I find myself pulling back, I re-examine my readiness or interest. For example, if you had asked me which of Fakir's intensive workshops I would be most likely to sign up for, I would have said the one on piercing. But when I attended his introductory piercing workshop, I found myself pulling away at least as many times as I moved forward. Even though my

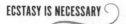

brain told me I was passionate about learning more about piercing, my body told me otherwise.

A direct, palpable, body-level attraction—feeling physically
pulled toward something—is the first indication that you're on
your way to an enthusiastic *yes*. You may feel that enthusiastic *yes*
immediately, or it may come to you days after your initial exposure to it.

What's been calling you lately?
What have you been finding yourself pulled closer to?

2. Consider the risk

In this step you ask yourself, "Is this really for me? Is it worth
my time, money, and/or emotional commitment? What effect will
making this choice have on the rest of my life and on those around
me? Is it in line with my highest values? Does it meet a particular
need? Is this an appropriate risk for me at this time? What are the
real dangers involved and what dangers am I imagining? What
conditions would need to be in place for me to consider following
through on this risk?"

Considering one's risk can be an emotional process, or it may
be more of a logistical one. In my case, the considerations for my
branding adventure were primarily logistical. I had to make time
in my schedule to fly across the country to attend the intensive
branding workshop. The primary challenge for me was whether I
could take time away from the writing of this book and still meet
my deadline. I planned this workshop months in advance, and I
suspected that by the time the workshop happened I would need
a break from writing. I knew I would appreciate a chance to drop
back into my body after months of primarily cerebral activity. I
also considered the fact that Fakir had recently turned 80 years
old and that the opportunity to study with him would not last

150

forever. To seal the deal, I decided to give myself the workshop as a birthday present, as my birthday was only a couple of days after the workshop ended.

A risk can be much more challenging if you are considering an activity with a significant emotional component. For example, what if you were contemplating having sex for the first time since your partner died? Or thinking about opening up your marriage/relationship to include sex and relationships with others? An appropriate risk is an erotic or ecstatic challenge that excites you—even to the point of occasional anxiety—as long as it does not paralyze you with fear and insecurity. Craft the risk so that it sits at your emotional Resilient Edge of Resistance.

One of the risk factors you may need to consider is whether or not this is an appropriate risk for you *at this time*. Maybe you want to try trance dancing, but it requires physical stamina and you're recovering from pneumonia. Or you'd like to take an intensive Tantric sex workshop, but you'd originally planned to go with the boyfriend you recently broke up with. In cases like these, you'll want to review the elements of building yourself a safe foundation in Chapter 3. Then see if you can gather enough of these elements to support you during this challenging time. If not, it might be better to postpone this particular risk, adventure, or challenge for a couple of months.

Another question to ask yourself when considering the appropriateness of a particular erotic risk is, "Why do I want to do this?" A satisfying answer to this question will help you answer a second question, "How do I want to do this?"

Are you taking this risk or challenge to prove something to yourself or to someone else? Have you been through a recent break up and want to prove your desirability? Are you trying to get the attention of a person or a group? Are you attempting to fill an emotional need that would be better met in therapy? These are not good reasons for taking an erotic risk. Ecstatic risks are best approached from the cleanest, clearest, and most compassionate part of your intuitive guidance system. That does not necessarily mean that your decision has to come out of an exclusively happy mood.

Fear, anger, and sadness make up three-quarters of your emotional guidance system. If any of these three emotions arise as you consider a new erotic challenge, it is not necessarily an indication that you shouldn't be pursuing the risk. Perhaps listening to the messages of this emotional mix will lead you to an enthusiastic *yes*.

For example, let's assume you are grieving the breakup of a recent relationship. Let's further assume that you have never been flogged before, but have been drawn to trying it. If your intention in being flogged is to receive a healing, being repeatedly flogged on the middle of your back at the heart chakra by a sensitive, skilled person can release oppressive emotions. It can leave you feeling cleansed. This intention of self-healing might be a completely appropriate motivation for risking an intense new experience.

However, if you are outwardly focused and all you want out of the flogging is to look adventurous, get the attention of the sexiest people in the room, and attract a slew of new sex partners, your experience of the actual flogging is likely to be disappointing. You may want to postpone this experience until you are motivated by a higher intention.

In short—it's not *what* you do but *why* you do it. The *why* informs the *how* and predicts the likelihood of an ecstatic result.

After you're clear on your motivation, do some research. Read how-to books or blogs or watch some videos to find out what others have experienced with the activity you're interested in exploring. Follow links from my website—and the websites of people you know and trust. As you do your research, pick your preferences. What about this activity turns you on the most? What, if any, aspect or variation of it turns you off? What props, tools, or techniques are required for maximum success in your activity?

The most significant part of my research had been watching Fakir's demonstration at the conference, but in making my final decision to attend the workshop, I went further. I talked to friends who experienced both giving and receiving brands. I read about different techniques and safeguards. I studied how to get the most artistically satisfying results.

The more you know, the more likely you are to be able to turn an erotic risk into an ecstatic opportunity.

If you think all this sounds overly calculated or lacking in spontaneity, trust me—there is plenty of spontaneity to be found in each present moment of a well-thought-out erotic risk.

There's no need to be overly ambitious in your scenarios. It is our intention to create experiences that are as mindful as possible, so plan on starting slowly and building up to an ecstatic adventure. You may not be able to play out your entire fantasy in one evening. For example, if you want to try anal sex for the first time, forgo the temptation to buy the big red dildo that looked so hot in the erotic video you watched with your lover, and buy the cute purple nitrile gloves and a luxurious lube instead.

Imagine an erotic or ecstatic risk you'd like to take.
What do you already know about the risk?
Where might you look for more information?
With whom might you want to talk?

3. Make a commitment

Now it's time to find your enthusiastic *yes*. An enthusiastic yes does not mean you have no fear, no apprehension, no questions. It simply means that you are excited enough—*enthusiastic* enough— to jump in and make a commitment. This is the step in which you send the e-mail, write the check, or make the phone call that says, "Yes, I'll be there."

That's just what I did. I filled out the registration form, wrote the check, and mailed them both. This certainly did not mean that I had no fears or reservations. I had just paid a substantial fee and made a commitment to fly across the country to learn how to permanently mark someone's skin with fire and hot metal. And

153

I'd agreed to be permanently marked myself, as the workshop was based on the premise that each participant would both brand and be branded. What if I sucked at it? What if I hated the feel of this particular form of fire? How was I going to explain this workshop to my friends? Sure, my friends in the BDSM world would understand—most of them, anyway—but this was *branding*. Even some kinky people draw the line at branding.

With all these fears and questions, why did I commit to going? Because the possibilities seemed so much bigger than the limitations of my fear. Because when I could quiet my nattering brain, which was desperately trying to protect me by insisting I be more sensible, I felt a boost of energy that transformed my tentative *yes* into a wildly enthusiastic *yes*.

This is probably a good moment to make a distinction and offer a warning. Be careful about allowing a tentative yes to become acquiescence. Acquiescence may feel like a yes, but is not really a yes at all—it's a cleverly disguised maybe. Acquiescence—often expressed as something along the lines of, "Well, okay, sure. I guess so. Uh yeah, well, okay. Why not?"—is a conditional, guarded position. When you're guarded you can't be fully present. You'll either be in the past, assessing whether or not that last touch was okay with you, or in the future, wondering if you're going to like what's coming next. By comparison, the enthusiastic yes—even when accompanied by some fear or doubt—brings you fully into the present moment.

The enthusiastic yes is very easy to recognize in the exploration of erotic ecstasy. It has that let's-do-it-right-now quality even if it's accompanied by some variation of "but I'm really scared I'll hate it."

My client, Kellie, had a baby in the past year and was still struggling to lose the excess weight. She had once enjoyed playing a sexy scene with her husband in which he was a patron at a strip club and she was a stripper. She would do a particularly hot and nasty strip number for him, and he would try and entice her into the back room for sex. "No, no," she would protest. "I can't! It's against the rules and I could get fired." This was his cue to tempt her with real money and real champagne. It was a seriously hot fantasy and he'd always managed to convince her to take the risk.

She was still drawn to this fantasy but was uncomfortable about playing it out at her current weight. She thought her husband wouldn't find her attractive and she imagined that it would ruin the fantasy for them in the future. I asked Kellie to take a breath and tell me what she was feeling in her body when she contemplated actually dancing the striptease. She replied that she felt excited, and she was getting turned on, but that she felt fear in her stomach. "So on a scale of one (drain) to ten (gain)," I asked, "is this thought an energy gain or an energy drain?" "It's about a seven," she reported.

"Good," I replied. "Let's see if we can raise the gain just a bit higher. What if you played the same scene, but changed the striptease to a lap dance. That would make it less of a visual performance, and more of a sensual experience for you both."

Now we had an enthusiastic yes—Kellie reported that her energy gain meter registered a nine! By lowering her fear of seeming unattractive to her husband, she found her enthusiastic yes.

It's often said that the journey of a thousand miles begins with one step. What is that one step for you?

4. Find support

This step does not fit in any particular sequential order in the process of erotic risk-taking. Finding support may be the first thing you do when you initially consider your risk. If not, from this point on, support from like-minded people is something that you'll likely want and appreciate in all the steps that follow.

In my case, I first turned to my partner Kate for support when I was debating whether or not I could spare the time to go to the workshop. She knows me well enough to know that I often use

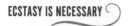

lack of time as an excuse when I'm not sure I'm making the right choice. Kate was able to remind me how excited I was when I saw the branding demonstration and how much this workshop was in line with both my values and my desires.

Next, I called Annie Sprinkle, who lives in San Francisco where the workshop would be held, and asked her if I could stay with her. I knew Annie would be the perfect support person—emotionally, artistically, and spiritually—during the weekend. The third person I called was my friend Sharrin Spector, a renowned body modification artist in the Bay Area, who first studied with Fakir some 18 years before. Sharrin owned her own body modification shop for many years and branding was one of the things she offered. Sharrin and I arranged to have dinner after the first day of workshop. I knew I could count on her for both moral and technical support.

Support can come from any number of sources—family, friends, and communities. Initially, you'll want to find people who have been there and done that, so to speak. Their experience does not have to be exactly the same as the one you're embarking upon, but it should be similar enough that they can relate to whatever risk you're taking. It's perfectly fine to share your desire for your particular ecstatic risk with people who are as unfamiliar and terrified as you are, but you'll want to make sure that the majority of your support comes either from experienced explorers, or from people who are as or more excited about your new adventure as you are.

There are many different communities—or tribes, as I like to think of them—and finding one's tribe or tribes is one of the most rewarding aspects of erotic exploration. People form communities around all sorts of ecstatic interests and pursuits. Within the larger groups there are smaller, special-interest groups of every possible description. Whether your passion is art, adventure, dance, spirituality, alternative relationships, sex, BDSM, or a host of others, you'll find a group dedicated to pursuing it to its fullest.

Finding an erotic community before the existence of the Internet was challenging. You either had to know someone who knew someone—or you'd have to subscribe to a special-interest magazine or newspaper. *Screw Magazine* in New York City listed all manner and description of sex clubs and sex parties. Magazines like *Screw* were extremely explicit and simply not to everyone's taste. Today, you can be extremely specific about your interests and receive information and invitations via e-mail exclusively for the activities you like. You can also be as anonymous as you like online. FetLife and Facebook are just two social networks featuring hundreds of erotic and ecstatic special-interest groups. There are also countless meet-up groups. All you have to do is type "meet up" and the name of your city or town into a search engine and you'll be able to search for local meet-up groups on virtually any topic, including the erotic and the ecstatic.

One of the easiest and most enjoyable ways of exploring a new interest and meeting members of a new tribe is to attend a workshop. Not only will you learn something new, you'll also meet like-minded folks in a situation where the focus is on learning and socializing, not entirely on sex and play. If you're looking for a relationship or a date, you certainly might find one, but since that's not the focus of the workshop, you won't feel pressured to do anything you're not ready for. Worldwide, there is an ever-increasing number of erotic events—often organized as conferences with a full schedule of workshops and social events over the course of a long weekend. At some of these events you can meet members of several different tribes, such as Tantrikas, kinky people, swingers, pagans, queers, and more. As your ecstatic explorations grow, you may find yourself a member of more than one tribe.

When we join and form new communities we feed our possibilities, instead of feeding our fears and doubts. Chances are you will meet someone who will tell you what an amazing time they have had pursuing the same passion you are nervous about exploring. Yet, when we first think of approaching a new group of people we can feel nervous about whether or not we will be accepted. Remember that everyone in that group was once the new person. My teaching partner, Chester, used to tell people who had just completed one of our adventurous erotic massage weekends,

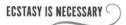
"Congratulations, you are now one of the people you were terrified of at the beginning of this weekend."

Why is the support of members of a community or tribe so important for ecstatic risk-taking? In our everyday lives, our harmless desires can easily be seen as weird, excessive, bizarre, or just plain wrong—or, on the other end of the spectrum—heroic, amazing, extraordinary, or exceptional. We all need to be part of a tribe in which we feel normal, average, and ordinary. Despite our culture's passion for celebrity and fame, we all need a community where we are just like everyone else. I've heard people ask, "Why do celebrities all hang out together" or "Why do all the presenters at spiritual or sexual events spend more time with each other than with attendees?" It's because they are receiving support from people engaged in similar challenges. They feel ordinary. It is far more frightening to be standing alone on the edge of a very high diving board than it is to be diving as part of a team, with all your teammates cheering for you in the pool below.

Whether you want to try pole-dancing, Tantric sex, erotic massage, trance dancing—or if you simply want to bring more consciousness and intimacy into your relationship—there's a group out there that would love to have you as a member.

You've now committed to taking an erotic risk.
You're on your way.
Whose hand would you like to hold?
Who would you like to have walking by your side?
What support do you need along the way?

5. Enjoy the anticipation

Anticipation is the phase that begins the moment after you make a commitment and extends to the moment in which you actually begin to take your erotic risk. This is the step in which you start to think or fantasize about what the experience might actually be like. Typically it is characterized by alternating degrees of fear and excitement.

In my case, my apprehension expressed itself—as it often does—as a fear that I could not afford to take the time away from my work. "Perhaps," I thought, "I should take the workshop later when I am not on deadline." In reality, I was still worried about whether or not I'd like branding. And of course all my worries were mixed with the thrill and excitement of finally giving myself permission to take one of Fakir's workshops.

In this stage we may wonder if we were right to have made the commitment in the first place. Perhaps we tried something like this once before and we weren't very good at it. Or perhaps this new challenge is completely outside our paradigm and therefore completely new and scary to us. Perhaps we are afraid that by trying this new activity we may lose our reputation, or the love and respect of someone we care about. Or maybe we're simply afraid of coming across as an idiot.

There is so much cultural shame around anything sexual or primal. That shame is often the first and most paralytic of the feelings that surface when we think about trying something new. Shame can manifest as: We are wrong for wanting to do this, we won't be good at it, people will laugh at us, and we will be humiliated.

This is a good time to remember the proverb about the two fighting wolves. I've modified the story to embrace our subject matter:

An ecstatic explorer tells a student, "A fight is going on inside me between two wolves. One wolf is shame, fear, guilt, regret, resentment, anger, envy, inferiority, and self-pity. The other wolf is joy, pleasure, self-acceptance, love, compassion, faith, sharing, truth, and passion. This same fight is going on inside you, and inside every other erotic explorer, too."

The student thought for a moment then asked the erotic explorer, "Which wolf will win?"

The erotic explorer replied: "The one you feed."

*Use bottom breathing (see Chapter 3) to enter into a
dialogue between your fear and your excitement.
Let your fear speak for three breaths.
Let your excitement speak for three breaths.
Continue for as long as they have something to say.*

6. Jump into the water

The day is here. The moment has almost arrived. This is when
the fear/excitement cycle is at its peak. For me, arriving a bit
early for a new experience helps me to feel calm and centered. I
arrived in San Francisco a day early so I could get plenty of rest
the night before the workshop. I got up early so I could take my
time and have a good breakfast. I arrived at the workshop space
a little early so I could meet the other participants, and have a
few minutes to chat with Fakir. All of this helped me to feel safer
and more prepared.

Do whatever you need to feel comfortable, prepared, and com-
petent. Did you bring water and a snack? If you're playing with a
new toy, have you practiced with it? For instance, if you are going
to play a scene with a strap-on dildo, have you tried on that new
harness and adjusted it in advance, so you can get in and out of
it quickly?

Resist the temptation to proceed with an erotic risk when
you're tired and hungry and/or distracted. Remember, you are not
being marched into battle. You are anticipating ecstasy. Ecstasy
requires mindfulness. The only place ecstasy exists is in each present moment. Therefore, *you* need to be physically and emotionally
present in the present moment.

When I got to Fakir's workshop room, I was eager but relaxed.
As I sat through the opening circle and heard everyone introduce
themselves, the old fears started to arise. "Oh dear," I thought.

"This is so new for me. Everyone else in this room is a tattoo artist or a piercer. They are all experienced body modification artists. I am certainly not in their league."

Fakir began to demonstrate the first branding technique—strike branding—the same technique I had seen him do at the conference in August. He placed a small, thin piece of metal in a vise grip and heated it in the flame of a propane torch until it was glowing orange. He then quickly and precisely touched the hot metal to a piece of corrugated cardboard—chosen because it would teach us how much pressure to apply. We were to burn through only the first thin layer of the cardboard. He then set us up in pairs at tables that had been covered with sheets of corrugated cardboard. It was our turn to try it.

Even though I knew I couldn't possibly hurt a piece of cardboard, my mind couldn't let go of the fact that I had no clue how to do this, yet by tomorrow I would be doing this on someone's skin. I was everywhere but in the present moment! I took a breath. I reminded myself, "Everything you're afraid of has either happened in the past or is something that you fear is going to happen in the future." All I had to do in this present moment was heat up a little piece of metal and touch it to the corrugated cardboard. That's all. Nothing more.

I inhaled and raised my vise grips. I waited until the little piece of metal glowed orange. I gently and quickly touched the glowing metal to the cardboard. Voilà! My first brand.

7. Release the need to be perfect

Whether we are picking up a condom, a dildo, a flogger, or a branding implement for the first time, it's hard to resist the temptation to want to be perfect immediately. Whether we're trying anal sex, Tantric sex, erotic massage, or cuddling, we somehow think we should instinctively know how to do it flawlessly the very first time.

Sometimes we actually can do something perfectly the first time we try it—but then we can't repeat it. I like to think of this as the universe's humorous way of dangling a chocolate mousse in front of us to keep us moving toward our goal and into our Totality of Possibilities. By giving us a taste of that chocolate mousse, we know that it's both attainable and worth attaining, so we keep moving forward.

My first nearly perfect brand on cardboard was followed by numerous less perfect strikes. I tried to remind myself that despite its potential in ritual and erotic transformation, the art of branding was in fact a skill. I had to keep practicing long enough to get the technique into my muscle memory, but our practice session had progressed into more refined skills. We were now focused not only on getting the metal hot enough and the depth of the strike right, but also on being able to strike a pre-drawn mark with perfect accuracy. Predictably, I did hit some marks perfectly and others much less perfectly.

No matter, I thought. *I'll have more time to practice later.* Besides, I knew I was going to be much better at the second type of branding—the one we were just about to learn: electrocautery. In electrocautery branding, you draw a design into the skin with a device that looks like a pen. Electrocautery works by introducing a high-frequency current through an electrode on the tip of the pen, causing it to become hot. It is used for branding because you can create patterns more intricate than you can using the traditional strike-branding method.

So, I sat down at a practice table outfitted with an electrocautery unit and a fresh piece of corrugated cardboard. One of Fakir's assistants, an expert in this type of branding, showed me how fast to move the pen and how deep the mark should be. With a pencil, I drew a curved line on the cardboard and proceeded to trace the line with the hot metal tip. It was a disaster! I was much worse at this than I was at strike branding. Try as I might, I could not produce either an even depth or a proper line. I tried again and again and again. No change. I asked Fakir for help. He gave me a couple of tips, and then confirmed what I already knew—I really wasn't getting this. He looked at me skeptically and told me to keep practicing.

It was the end of the first session. We were now halfway through the workshop. I felt I had no hope of mastering this in one more day. I was being unreasonably hard on myself, but I knew there was some key piece to this that I was missing. I had no idea what it was or how I could change it. I was exhausted, demoralized, and humiliated. I saw myself through the eyes of my ego: me and my experience were separate from everyone else and their experience. It never occurred to me that others leaving the workshop probably felt the same way. Lucky for me, I was meeting my friend Sharrin Spector for dinner.

Sharrin saw at once that things had not gone as well as they might have. "Listen," she said, "I know that you're going to be *really* good at this. You're a natural. In fact, you're going to enjoy electrocautery a lot more than strike branding. I'll bet you the price of a dinner that electrocautery is the branding technique that you'll wind up using all the time after you leave here."

Sharrin dug in her bag and pulled out a chunky marker, roughly the size of the electrocautery pen. "Show me how you were holding the pen today," she said. I did. "Well, that's part of the problem," said Sharrin. "Try holding it exactly like a pen. Pretend you're going to draw a line really slowly. That's good! Okay, now tomorrow morning before you go back to the workshop, go to the grocery store and buy yourself a nectarine. Practice on that—it's much more like skin. You'll be amazed at the difference."

Then Sharrin and her partner, Pat, proceeded to buy me a magnificent dinner and a couple of glasses of wine after which I was more inclined to let tomorrow take care of itself.

Releasing the need to be perfect is an essential step in erotic risk-taking.

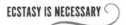

Where does your perfectionist streak
show itself most frequently?
Where has it or might it show up in the
process of your erotic risk-taking?
Recall the times you have successfully
released your need to be perfect.
Recall the ways in which you have successfully
released your need to be perfect.

8. Rest and regroup.

When something goes wrong in a first attempt at a new endeavor, I advocate the scream-and-shout response. Feel your feelings. Whether you're feeling upset, embarrassed, angry, humiliated, or stupid, let it out. No matter how miserably things seem to have gone, talking them out will start to soften the edges. Whether it's hearing the story as you're telling it, or seeing the look in your supportive friends' eyes as they hear it, the extreme emotions will start to shift. A glimmer of perspective and hope will appear—truly, it will.

After my bad day branding and my great meal with Sharrin, I went home to Annie's place. Some 20 years earlier, it was Annie who had convinced me that I was an artist in my own right and not just a manager and producer of other artists' work. To this day I credit Annie for the recovery of my artistic soul. That evening she listened, she sympathized, and she told me that she knew tomorrow would be different. Then she distracted me by asking me to help her with an art project she was working on. Despite all my accumulated artistic doubts, I was able to be of some help, which left me feeling like I'd ended the day with at least some small win.

Do not go to sleep on a defeat. Create a win for yourself, no matter how small.

Even if it's just vacuuming the cat hair off your carpet, or finishing a sink full of dishes, or answering one overdue e-mail—go to sleep knowing that you successfully accomplished something.

9. Try, try again . . . or don't.

It is more difficult to muster courage when you've had a taste of failure. As Rick Hanson points out in his book *Buddha's Brain*, the human brain is wired to detect trouble far more quickly than happiness or peace—a holdover from our primitive past when such wiring was necessary for survival. In addition, negative events have more impact than positive ones—people will do more to avoid a loss than to acquire a comparable gain. So, whenever something doesn't work out well the first time, we have a tendency to believe that it won't work out the next time, even though statistics have proven that things actually turn out well or neutral more often than they turn out badly.

When our erotic risk results in anything less than an immediate ecstatic payoff, our brains send out a warning, leading us to believe that the risk we've chosen to take is too dangerous or not worth pursuing. After all, we reason, how can this activity ever be ecstatic when I can't even manage to make it pleasant? This is the time for some quiet introspection. Perhaps you've discovered that the reason the risk you took didn't work out is because the activity is really not right for you. Or you just didn't like it. Or you didn't like the people who were participating. You are under no obligation to try this activity again if you don't want to. Trust your instincts.

If your scene went wrong and someone else is involved, be sure to check in with them as soon as you can. Whether you ever want to play with this person again or not, you owe it to yourself and to them to find some completion, perspective, and peace around the situation.

If you do want to take the risk again, ask yourself: What do I need to do differently this time? Do I need a different setting or a different partner? What do I know now that I did not know first time I tried this? How might I change my thinking about this?

Me? I needed a nectarine. I got up extra early and went to the local supermarket where I was dismayed to find that nectarines weren't in season. I squeezed my way through the fruit section feeling for anything that vaguely resembled a nectarine. I found a ripe mango. *Oh great!* I thought. *A smelly tropical fruit—perfect for me!* But, what could I do? I was desperate. I bought it, along with a pack of peppermint chewing gum, in hopes that the mint would overpower the smell of the mango.

Deep in my being I knew that this mango was the secret to my artistic success. I arrived at the workshop space early, to practice. I did not discuss or explain my mango. I merely asked if I could practice with the electrocautery unit. Fakir looked at me, then my mango, then me again, and dubiously said yes. I sat down and drew an attractive design on my mango, incorporating both straight lines and curvy lines. I fired up my electrocautery pen. I took a deep breath and touched the orange-hot tip to the mango. It sliced through it like—well, like it was a mango. It was instantly easy. My line was perfect and the depth was nearly perfectly even. I continued. I drew another design, more complex this time. Sharrin had been so right. Not only was this easy, this was delicious good fun.

A couple of my classmates came over to see what I was doing. They confessed that they were having a little trouble with the electrocautery unit themselves and also needed to practice. I asked them if they'd like to practice on my mango. One young woman looked so grateful and so relieved. She sat down and voilà! She, too, experienced instant success on the mango.

This one little win changed everything. My intuition had been right. Yes, yesterday had been awful, but that was not failure—that was inexperience. I was actually *talented* at this! I was not going to permanently disfigure someone today—I was going to help give them a body modification they, and I, could be proud of.

10. Surrender and enjoy.

This step could also be called "let go and let bliss." You are finally standing at the top of the hill. Having climbed to this height, all it takes is one more breath. All you need to do is press forward till you feel your fear push back just a bit. There it is—your Resilient Edge of Risk. You're just where you need to be: ready to let go and fly.

I was now giddy with relief and enthusiasm. I knew that with proper supervision I could actually follow a line drawn on someone's skin and create a brand safely and properly. This feeling of confidence as a brander allowed me to see the ecstatic possibilities of being a brandee. I knew that breathing could transform a painful process into a transformative ecstatic experience. As a giver, I use this breath-based sensation-processing technique: always move on an exhale. I had learned this years before and it has never let me down. Whether the activity was thrusting during sex or delivering a sexy spanking, the receiver was best able to process a sensation when they were exhaling. How do you know exactly when someone is exhaling? You breathe with them.

I was relieved to discover that none of us had to complete an entire brand by ourselves. At least two of us would participate in the creation of any one design. I did not offer to pick up a branding implement during the first brand. It was my hope that by audibly setting up a conscious rhythmic breath, both the branders and the receivers would have an easier time. Sure enough, as soon as everyone in the room was breathing together I could feel the level of fear and anxiousness in the room diminish and see the quality and ease of the branding increase. When the first brand was finished, we divided into small teams. It was now my turn to brand. The design drawn on my classmate's leg had both curved and straight lines, which would be made permanent with electrocautery. One of the instructors began the brand, reminding us how fast and deep to go, and then it was my turn. I picked up the pen and breathed into the feeling of confidence and ease I remembered from my session with the mango. I touched the orange hot tip to skin. It was thrilling! I was calm. I was focused. I was simultaneously anchored to the ground and flying around the room in triumph.

After a while, I passed off the electrocautery pen to the classmate who would complete this brand, and I moved on to another table where Fakir was supervising a classmate. She was working on a foot-long Tree of Life design that ran up another classmate's hip and side. The young woman receiving the brand was in an endorphin trance. You would've thought that we were simply drawing on her side with magic markers instead of with fire. This design was a delightful artistic challenge, combining both thick and thin lines. Fakir looked at me with ambivalence, recalling my struggles of the day before. He asked if I felt up to working on this design. I looked at him with utter calm assurance. "Oh yes," I said.

I greeted my classmate on the table, established a conscious breath between the two of us, and proceeded to get lost in the magical tree that was growing up her body. I was in bliss and I was facilitating another's bliss. I had not felt so good in weeks. I felt as one with my skill, my classmates, and the process of life.

I was the last to receive a brand. I had chosen a simple line drawing that combined a valentine heart with a spiral. For me this mark symbolized love, compassion, spiritual growth, and rebirth. Seth, our teaching assistant in electrocautery, began the brand. I took a few a deep breaths and as the pen touched my skin, I sailed into a gigglegasm. Branding felt like nothing I had ever experienced before. It plugged me into the source of all energy. The sensation of being branded was like a liquid fire—not painful but warm and intense. Grin (yes, that's his name) was one of the other teaching assistants. We had become friends over the course of the weekend. He leaned over me and started whispering a beautiful and profound heart meditation into my ear. Grin took me on a journey through every realm of heart-filled experience: loving hearts, compassionate hearts, broken hearts, and hearts cracked open. My gigglegasms were followed by crygasms and screamgasms, then back to gigglegasms. Some-where in the middle of the journey I was aware that Fakir had picked up the pen and was finishing the other side of the heart. *I let go and let ecstasy.* It was a perfect experience. When I got off the massage table, I felt like I was capable of containing all the love in the universe.

Now let's be real—you do not have to learn how to brand or be willing to be branded in order to find this kind of fulfill-ment. Your erotic/ecstatic risk might be as simple as asking some-one you've been secretly admiring out to dinner. Or as gentle as receiving an erotic massage after which you can fall into a soft bed without being expected to reciprocate. Or as quiet as a week alone in a cabin deep in the woods. Any erotic or ecstatic risk you wish to take can carry you into these realms. As with most everything in life, it's not what you do, but why you do it, and how you do it that matters. Ecstatic experiences do not stop with the cessation of the stimulus that brought you to a peak. In fact, that's often when the bliss begins. Surrendering into the afterglow of a peak experi-ence will produce its own rewards and further transformation. It can also go on for hours. Enjoy the journey. Celebrate! Meditate! Laugh! Cry! Scream! Tweet it! Fall into a big puddle of ecstatic relief. Surrender. You've worked hard to get here. Don't miss a mo-ment of the bliss.

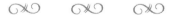

CHAPTER 6

The Language of Ecstasy

Thus far I have spoken about numerous possible impediments to ecstasy and ways to avoid, prevent, or transform these obstacles. As many of us have learned through experience, whether we fly high—or crash and burn—in the pursuit of our ecstatic endeavors is largely dependent on the effectiveness of our communication.

Communication is a basic human need and a fundamental social process. However—as with sex—different people communicate differently. Just as with sex, how to communicate, when to do it, how often to do it, how deeply to do it, with whom to do it, and with what expectation—is all open for discovery and discussion.

At best, the words "communicate" and "communication" are an umbrella term for a vast array of methods by which human beings and other life forms attempt to relate to each other. At worst, these two words have become so generalized, unspecific, and overused that they have almost been drained of meaning. Attached modifiers, such as "open" and "honest" are equally vague. For example, which of the many definitions of the word "open"

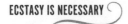

might apply to communication? And if the communication were not open, to whom would it be closed? The word "honest" is not much more helpful. Do we really want blunt honesty in all our speaking? Wouldn't that create at least as many problems as it might solve?

I know I am not the only one for whom phrases such as "open, honest communication" elicits a "get me out of here" response second only to that of the dreaded "We need to talk . . ." In order for our communication to support us in our quest for ecstatic experience, we need to become more deliberate and more precise in our language, and we need to approach communication of all types—including nonverbal—with conscious intention.

This chapter contains two parts. In the first part you'll become more aware of how you communicate now. You'll learn creative uses of language—verbal and nonverbal—and discover how to communicate effectively with someone whose style of speaking is different from yours. You will discover effective ways to ask for what you want and learn how to speak up when something isn't working for you. You'll also get to practice the art of listening more deeply. In the second part of the chapter, you'll learn how to use language to create fulfilling erotic and ecstatic connections and encounters.

Speaking with Conscious Intention

In Chapter 2, I asked you: *Why do you do sex—what do you get out of it? What's the delight?* Let's ask the same questions about communication: *Why do you communicate?*

Here are a few examples, just to get you thinking:

- To amuse, delight, or entertain

- To change someone's mind or to convince them of something

- To comfort/soothe or to ask for comfort/soothing

- To excite or enthuse

- To explain or to ask for explanation

- To get someone to behave differently

- To give or to get love

- To be heard and understood

- To make friends

- To name something, to differentiate one thing from another

- To negotiate, to reach an agreement

- To be noticed

- To turn someone on or to seduce them

- And—as my friend Eric Wunderman reminded me—to get the salt from one end of the dinner table to the other

There is nothing inherently wrong with any communication intention—with, of course, the exceptions of intentions to bully, intimidate, and harm. Short of that, there is nothing wrong in trying to persuade someone to see things our way. Is it inappropriate, for instance, to try to convince a recovering addict to take the medicinal dose of morphine that will help save their life? Or to speak with the intention of turning someone on? Too often, however, we are unaware of our intention when we are speaking. We try to convince someone of something "for their own good," when in fact, our actual intention is to get them to do something for *our* own good.

When everyone agrees, or mostly agrees, with each other, it is easy to hold a positive intention for a conversation. Whenever we feel fear—whatever its specific nature—our positive intentions can quickly fly out the window. Speaking from personal experience,

I can recall countless conversations in which my sole intention was to get out of the room as quickly as possible. This is hardly an intention likely to lead to an ecstatic conclusion.

When a conversation triggers our fight-or-flight response, our intentions are reduced to "I've gotta win this!" or "Goddess, please let me survive this." Either of these is a good indication that the intention we held when we entered the conversation was probably not clear enough or positive enough. Perhaps we were thinking, *I have the perfect argument to make them see that I am right,* or *I've worked out just the right way to tell them that I don't want to do what they want me to do—without getting them mad at me.*

In situations where we know in advance that we are facing a potentially difficult conversation with one or more people, it pays to set an intention that includes a desire for an outcome that is for everyone's highest good. There is nothing wrong with focusing on an outcome you hope to achieve. But, instead of speaking solely with the intention of convincing someone to do something differently, what if we were to approach the conversation . . .

. . . with a sense of curiosity? What if our intention was to discover something new about the speaker?

. . . assuming that the person to whom we were speaking wished us enormous quantities of joy, pleasure, and happiness?

. . . with the intention of reducing shame and feelings of unworthiness in ourselves and others?

How would that change our verbal language? Or body language? Our listening? The outcome of the conversation?

Recall a conversation that you recently had or imagine one that you're about to have. What is/was your initial intention for the conversation? What higher intention would be/would have been a good companion to your original intention?

There are many good resources on effective and compassionate communication, and I'll talk about some of them later. Before we discuss any of the how-to's, let's prioritize the setting of clear intentions. Let's practice making space alongside our initial intention—whether it's to convince, amuse, or seduce—to include a *higher* intention. If you find it difficult to think of a specific higher intention you can always use this affirmation: "May the outcome of this conversation be for the highest good and greatest happiness of all concerned."

Say It in Plain Language

We humans have been inventing new languages from the moment we learned to speak. As we migrated into new territories and met other humans, our languages adapted, expanded, and combined until today, there are somewhere between 3,000 and 10,000 living languages. According to Ethnologue (www.ethnologue.org), 6,909 is thought to be the likely number. This does not include the many dialects spoken within these languages. Nor does this include the numerous jargon and slang sub-languages spoken in each tongue.

You've probably seen a version of this skit countless times: A patient asks a doctor for a diagnosis. The doctor rattles off a completely incomprehensible two minutes of Latin/medical mumbojumbo. When the doctor finally stops talking, the patient asks, "Hey, doc, can you say that in English?" The doctor replies, "You have the flu." It's an old joke. But let's look at it a new way. Let's look at the intention of each of the speakers.

The patient's intention was to get information about their health. Were they going to die from this ailment, they wondered? Could they get back to work next week? The doctor's intention might have been to give the patient complete and precise information. The doctor's intention could also have been to impress the patient by sounding as authoritative as possible. In any event, no one's intention could be fulfilled until both parties were speaking and hearing the same language.

Every social group, religion, school, and profession has its own jargon—a particular subset of the native language. In many cases this includes a unique style of speaking—a rhythm, a cadence, or a rhyme, for example—as well as the use of specific words. As long as everyone in the conversation speaks the language, all is well. If, for example, New Age people are sharing in healing circles while corporate people are negotiating in meeting rooms, everyone has a fairly good chance of being understood. However, imagine the scene if they were all to sit down in one room and try to communicate using only their tribal languages.

Here's a short list of some of these specialized sub-languages: Medical speak, tech talk, corporate speak, therapy speak, religious speak (all denominations), New Age speak, art (including theatre, dance, music, etc.) speak, academic speak, 12-step speak, yoga speak, legalese, finance speak, political speak, Internet and texting speak, Star Trek speak, and twin speak—that secret language only understood between a pair of twins. Then of course there's slang, as in hip-hop slang, beatnik slang, hippie slang, cockney rhyming slang, and more.

Make a list of all the different "languages" you speak.
How many of these do you think are easily understood by . . .
Your lover? Your family? Your best friend? Your co-workers?
Think of at least one instance where you were left feeling
baffled, angry, or excluded when someone used their
"language" and you had no idea what was being said.

One function of jargon is to intentionally distinguish members of a group from non-members. This gives the members a sense of solidarity and empowerment. But often things go too far and even the initiated don't understand what is being said. My friend Ingrid Geronimo offers a great example:

> If you go from one corporate job to another, you ultimately wind up with a language gap—you have to learn a whole new set of acronyms or nomenclature. This can cause you to feel like you're so far behind the game that you question whether you really know what you thought you knew when you got hired. On top of all this, everyone assumes you know what they're talking about because you're in the same industry.

Joining a group with a new tribal language can be exciting. We all want to be better understood and to feel that we belong, and this new language appears to be authentic and effective at communicating the values, needs, and desires of the group. When the language is new and fresh to us, we speak our new sub-language with intention and precision. However, over time, our new language can grow stale and may dissolve into platitudes, catchphrases, and obscure references.

One common feature of tribal speak is the use of three or four or five words—or three- or four- or five-syllable words—where one or two words would suffice. Initially our intentions are good. More words, bigger words, or made-up words appear to make our speaking more precise, but as Lubyanka observed in her blog at ladylubyanka.wordpress.com:

> My experience of flouncy communication is that it tends to be an indirect, unhelpful, inflammatory, unresponsive, and obscure way to express something like "I'm unhappy with that and would rather it were like this."

Tribal speech, especially when used outside of the tribe, is usually an indirect way of speaking. For example, if you're apprehensive about saying to your partner "I hated that sex party and I never want to go near anything like it again," you might borrow language from your healing and meditation group and say, "I found the energy a bit negative and I did not feel much of a heart connection with anyone there." Your partner, hearing this, may not be angry with you, but they also probably have no clue that you never want to go to a party like that again. They might logically assume that on some future evening the energy will be more positive, the crowd friendlier, and you'll likely meet new people with whom you'll feel more of a connection. The whole situation you're trying to avoid is likely to arise again sometime soon.

The use of carefully worded tribal speak is also a great way to avoid answering a direct question. Let's imagine that someone you don't much like asks if you would like to have a relationship with them. Your inner voice is loudly screaming "No! I would rather stick needles in my eyes!" However, the polite, placating part of you answers with a long, fluffy explanation about why the circumstances of your job leave you with no time for personal growth and exploration and that you desperately need some private space and alone time. Would you wonder why they keep texting you, asking if the pressure of your job has eased up and if you now have time?

Another reason we dilute our language—and thus its meaning—is to give ourselves wiggle room. Obscure speech is a way of sticking our toe in the water to gauge the temperature of someone's reaction before we dare to step in and speak plainly. Unfortunately, when we begin a conversation with diluted language, we may find it difficult to break the pattern of obscure speech and talk more explicitly about the issue later.

Whether your intention is to convey an idea, a feeling, or a plea, the language you choose to deliver your message will determine how accurately and easily your message is received.

*Recall a time in which you assumed that someone under-
stood you, only to find out later that they had completely
missed or misunderstood what you were trying to say.
Recall a time when you did not ask for
clarification when you needed it.*

Language Is More than Words

Growing up in the theatre, I quickly learned that the playwright's
words were only a starting point in the exchange between the ac-
tors and the audience. Arthur Laurents—the author of the books of
musicals such as *West Side Story* and *Gypsy*—said it well: "plays are
emotions"—not simply words strung together. As a theatre artist,
it was my job to make all the other languages of theatre—acting,
directing, scenery lighting, costumes, sound, music, and dancing—align with, support, and illuminate the playwright's message.
I learned that no matter how clear and profound the words, if
they were spoken with the inappropriate intent, or surrounded
by shoddy production values, the audience would not hear the
message. Often when things were feeling stale or inauthentic in
rehearsal, we would put down the script and play a scene without
words. We might mime or dance or gesticulate—whatever it took
to communicate our character's message to other characters and
to the audience.

Like plays, *relationships are emotions*. Sometimes no matter
how hard we try, and no matter how understanding our partner(s)
might be, we simply can't put what we feel into words. This is
when we need to remember that language and communication
take many forms. If you can't describe what you feel, try drawing the feeling. Pick up some crayons and a blank piece of paper
and let your hand move across the page. You don't have to draw

anything representational—you can just draw an abstract expression of your feelings. In the event that you find yourself in tears, or feel so angry that you break your crayons, just breathe and keep drawing. When you finish the first drawing, start a second. Let this new drawing represent the way you would *like* to feel.

When you finish your drawings, if you feel that the drawings effectively communicate your feelings—or that they might provide a starting place for that communication—you can share them with your partner. Or, you can take a break—walk around the block or have a cup of tea in the garden. Notice if you feel clearer and more able to identify your feelings. If so, you can try putting those feelings into words in your journal. Often our intentions become clearer when we write before we speak. When you feel that your words match your feelings, you can then share them with your friend or partner.

You can also dance or sing your way into your feelings. Turn on some music, close your eyes, and let loose. As was the case with your drawings, you do not have to share your song or dance with the person you're trying to communicate with, but you can if you think it will help.

There are many other forms of communication, which are either nonverbal, or that place words secondary to action. Dr. Gary Chapman, a marriage counselor and author of *The Five Love Languages*, observed that everyone he counseled had a "love language." These love languages were distinct preferences in the way people expressed their love and preferred to receive love from others.

The five love languages are:

1. *Words of Affirmation:* If this is your love language, you want to hear how much someone loves you and why. Unsolicited compliments from someone you love mean the world to you.

2. *Quality Time:* If this is your love language, you feel loved when you have your lover's full, undivided attention.

3. *Receiving Gifts:* If this is your love language, you appreciate the love and effort behind thoughtful, meaningful gifts.

4. *Acts of Service:* If this is your love language, you feel loved and appreciated when your lover says, "Let me do that for you."

5. *Physical Touch:* If this is your love language, you feel loved when someone is physically present and accessible, and shows their love with hugs, holding hands, thoughtful touches, etc. It is not limited to sexual or sensual touch.

Love languages are just one way of expressing the different ways in which we prefer to give and receive love and affection. Another way of expressing these differences is with the sensory preferences model used in Neuro-Linguistic Programming, or NLP. We each have a sense through which we prefer to take in and process the information we receive from the world around us. Some people get their information through pictures and images, others through sounds. Still others perceive chiefly through physical sensations. The preference we use when we process information—be it sight, sound, touch, smell, or taste—is likely to be our preference in sensual and erotic relating as well.

When we learn to speak each other's preferred language of love, our loved ones receive the message of love in the way that they can most easily understand and appreciate it. Relationships may improve dramatically with just this single awareness.

Learning to speak any of the various languages of love does not have to be difficult or time-consuming. It's easy and works like this: *Ignore* the Golden Rule. Do *not* do unto others as *you* would have them do unto *you*. Instead, follow the Platinum Rule: Do unto others the way *they* would have you do unto *them*.

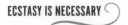

The Language of Breath

I loved the National Theatre of Great Britain's production of *War Horse*. It is a story of World War I told through the eyes of a horse named Joey, who was sent to the front at the beginning of the war. Joey is played by an intricate life-size puppet made of wood, wires, and translucent brown fabric. As a fully-grown horse, Joey is animated by three puppeteers: two stand inside his body, and the puppeteer who animates his head stands outside. When we first see Joey in the opening scene of the play, he is a young foal. Because this puppet is so small, the three puppeteers must stand alongside him to animate him. Our first impression is of a puppet and three puppeteers. Nonetheless, we empathize with this young foal taking his first steps. How? When Joey first enters, he frolics downstage, looks at us, and holds perfectly still. The only movement and sound is of his breathing. Nothing else. Just breath. We instinctively begin to breathe along with him. By the second or third breath, we are already empathizing with Joey. The breath creates our bond with him—the three puppeteers seem to vanish. This conversation with breath is used consistently throughout the nearly three-hour-long play. Whenever the puppeteers want to express an emotion they say it first with breath, then support it with other appropriate equine body language.

It works exactly the same way with people and in real life. We can "hear" each other through our breath. We can understand one another's feelings through our breath. We may intuit someone's motivation for their actions through their breath. When we breathe with someone, we have a visceral sense of the way they are feeling.

Conscious Naming

When we name something, we use language to differentiate it from something else. When we release an old name and take on a new one, we make a conscious shift into a new identity. It's like opening your journal and writing a title on the top of an empty page. This title will have a substantial influence over the nature and content of what follows on that page. It is much the same way when you name a person or a relationship. When you call yourself *married* as opposed to *single*, for example, the change in the name of the relationship changes that relationship. The change is even deeper if you choose to take your partner's last name, or to combine your last names. When we change our name or the name of our relationship, we are communicating to the outside world that we have a new identity.

Relationships and relationship names can be far more varied and creative than the commonly used *single, married, boyfriend, girlfriend, husband,* and *wife*. I asked a random sampling of people at a yearly conference I attend to tell me the names that they used to refer to a significant other. These are not pet names. These are names that real, live people use to identify their relationship or their significant other. Here are just some of their answers:

Beloved	Gnome	Pony
Boss	Houseboy	Primary partner
Boulder	Husband	Princess
Boyfriend	Imzadi	Puppy
Co-conspirator	Life partner	Puppy cat
Co-explorers	Lover or Lovers	Queen/knight
Cohort	Master	Secondary partner
Consort	Master/slave	Service human
Daddy/boi or Daddy/boy	Mommy/boi	Significant other
	My someone	Sir
Delight	Owner	Slave
Fellow journeyer	Paramour	Slaveboy
Friend	Partner or Partners	Slutling
Gentleman and Lady friends	Partner in crime	Soul mate
	Play partner	Spoose
Girl	Playmate	Wife
Girlfriend		

Keep in mind, these are not simply endearments such as *honey*, *sweetie*, or *baby*. These are actual *identities*. Boggles the mind, doesn't it? Since all these names represent different identities, it follows that all these relationships are unique. Each of these relationships was named to honor the essence of the specific connection between two or more people in the relationship. Conversely, each relationship has developed along a certain path *because of its name*.

One reason to consciously name relationships is to differentiate one relationship from another. Some of the people who shared with me their names for relationships are non-monogamous. They wanted a separate name for each of several partners and relationships. In other cases, some monogamous people had divorced a husband or a wife and now preferred to name and create some other kind of erotic partnering.

Another reason to consciously name is to allow us to circumvent negative associations we may have to commonly used words. For example, words such as *marriage*, *family*, and *community* are generally thought to be words that describe positive, loving institutions. However, if your family of origin kicked you out of the house for being gay, or you recently went through an expensive, acrimonious divorce, or if your political or sexual leanings have made you a pariah in your community, you may not feel all warm and fuzzy when you hear the words *family*, *marriage*, or *community*. It's a good idea to find out how the person you're talking to feels about a certain word or term before assuming that its consistent use will be welcomed and appreciated.

Differences in the naming of relations and relationships illustrate and reflect other values and preferences as well. Some people feel safe and cared for when there is a strong tangible connection between all the members of a particular network—be that professional, social, familial, or erotic. Other people feel safe and respected when strong boundaries and explicit agreements are in place. Unsurprisingly, these different types of folks use different names for similar relationships. For example, I have a friend who has referred to the man her mother married after divorcing her father as *stepfather* from the day their engagement was announced.

Another friend has referred to her mother's second husband as *my mother's husband* for more than 20 years.

Gender is becoming increasingly more fluid. People of blended or indeterminate gender can be found in ever-increasing numbers all over the world. If you are not sure of someone's gender, it is perfectly proper to politely ask, "Excuse me, which pronoun do you prefer?" or "What's your pronoun of choice?" If you're not comfortable asking either of these, simply avoid pronouns altogether and simply refer to them by their name. "They" is once again becoming increasingly accepted as a third-person singular, gender-free pronoun.

Let me be clear. I am not implying that you are expected to read everyone's mind and take into account every possible linguistic sensitivity anyone might have. That would be taking political correctness to an excruciating extreme. Rather, it is up to each of us to speak up if someone is using a word to describe us or our relationships that annoys, angers, hurts, or offends us—or is simply not quite the right fit. If we want others to follow the Platinum Rule, it's our responsibility to tell them what we want, and to do so as soon as we can. Postponing a correction can lead to serious and painful misunderstandings down the road.

Different Styles of Communication

Humans communicate in a variety of styles. Many of the styles in which people communicate result in easy, delightful, amusing, and erotic conversations. But we also communicate with the intention of getting what we want and in the hopes of getting something to change. It is in these situations when we are most likely to feel the effects of our different styles of communication.

People approach negotiation and/or conflict resolution—both personal and professional—in different ways. Our unique style of communication is not simply a preference—it's more like a default, or a template. We use our preferred communication style unconsciously. There is nothing inherently wrong with any style of communication. The confusion arises when our style either

185

doesn't match or is not compatible with the style of the person with whom we're talking.

When we become more conscious of our default style of communication and learn to recognize the default style of the people we are communicating with, we can expand and adapt our speaking and our listening. Our style of communication even offers clues as to what we need as part of any agreement.

Communication styles are not arbitrary or accidental. They are all based upon the speaker's genuine needs. Each person *needs* something out of an exchange in order for a negotiation process to feel successful and complete. Whether it's a profit, a good feeling, or the certainty that the right thing was done, if each speaker's needs are not met, the conversation will probably not lead to a lasting agreement.

Let's take a look at some common styles of communication to see how style and need inform each other:

Preferred Style	Key Phrase	Description
Legal or business	Let's make a deal.	These people want to come to an agreement by which everyone can abide. They need to make a deal in which they can be reasonably assured of realizing some sort of return on their investment of time, love, money, etc.
Mechanical or scientific	Let's figure out how this will work.	These people need to understand the mechanics of the situation. They like to break things down into their individual component parts, observe how those parts function individually and as a unit, then put them back together in some workable way.

Preferred Style	Key Phrase	Description
Therapeutic or psychological	Let's heal this.	These people want to analyze the situation for the purpose of healing the wound. They are concerned with feelings and emotions. They are less concerned with whether a solution is profitable or workable, than whether everyone feels good about it.
Academic or theoretical	Let's think this through.	These people want to know how this situation could be informed by hypothetical and theoretical thinking. They want to examine all the data and test a law or theorem. They need step-by-step proof based on established knowledge and theories.
Military or hierarchical	Let's fight it out.	These people need a clear win. Right and wrong is important to them. They are willing to fight long and hard for what they believe.
Medical or surgical	Let's find a cure.	These people need to solve the problem by finding something that will alleviate the symptoms or eliminate the cause and thereby stop the problem from hurting or spreading.
Artistic or entertaining	Let's imagine.	These people want to use their creativity. They need to see the situation in a new light and try something different. They are likely to ask, "How can we make this the most fun?"
Judicial	Let's obey the law.	These people need to find a just solution based upon the law, customs, or rules of a community or tribe. Their primary concern is whether a solution is fair and equitable according to those laws, customs, or rules.

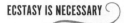
Preferred Style	Key Phrase	Description
Anarchistic	Let's smash the system.	These people are interested in ignoring or breaking the rules that restrict them and need to see just how far outside the lines they can color.
Buddhist or Taoist	There is no problem.	This is the path of Radical Acceptance. These people are equally comfortable accepting the situation as it is, or walking away in peace.

As you can see, no matter which of the above styles people prefer, they each require a particular need to be met in the course of discussion or negotiation in order to feel satisfied. A person who needs to find a just and fair solution which satisfies the rules of a certain organization or community would have a hard time getting that need met when negotiating with an anarchist who needs to find a solution that flaunts those same laws. An academic who needs proof based on established knowledge and theories might find it challenging to get what they need while trying to satisfy an artist who needs an innovative, entertaining solution.

The practice of Radical Acceptance can build a bridge over stylistic gaps. When we accept that a situation is the way it is without expectation that the essential facts will change, it is easier to focus on the needs behind the styles of communication.

For example:

The situation: Pamela and her partner, Casey, have been in a monogamous relationship for five years. Recently, Pamela has wanted to explore her submissive side and has been longing to find a dominant play partner, as Casey is not interested in dominating Pamela or anyone else. Pamela met Alexis, a potential play partner, online and has had a coffee date with Alexis (with Casey's knowledge). Pamela would now like to schedule a play date with her new friend.

What's not going to change—or at least not anytime soon: Casey is not interested in exploring domination. Pamela's interest in exploring her submissive side is not going to go away.

The communication styles involved: Pamela's communication style is therapeutic/psychological. Whatever the outcome, Pamela needs to know that everyone feels good about it. Casey's style is legal/business. Casey wants to come to an agreement by which everyone can profit.

Can these needs be met? Yes! Casey has no problem with Pamela exploring submission with Alexis so long as everyone agrees to a few rules: Pamela can play with Alexis no more than once every two weeks. There must be no kissing and no genital sex. In exchange, Casey wants to spend one afternoon or evening a week with Pamela with no agenda or outside distractions. Casey's love language is quality time, so the "profit" Casey realizes from this arrangement is uninterrupted time with Pamela.

Pamela can agree to these conditions, but only if she knows that Casey truly feels okay about opening up their relationship to accommodate her new interest. Casey assures her, not only verbally, but also by speaking Pamela's love language, touch: Casey holds her hand and hugs her close. Any discussion of a sensitive issue such as opening up a relationship could turn into a painful, potentially relationship-ending, screaming match. But by practicing Radical Acceptance and being aware of—and sensitive to—the needs behind our different styles of communication, we can bring new levels of consciousness into our negotiations.

Most of us have one or more secondary styles of communication in addition to our primary style. For example, a person with a medical/surgical style who wants to find a cure that will eliminate the problem might also prefer the solution to be new and creative. A person with an academic/theoretical style, who wants proof based on established theories, might also care that everyone involved feels good about the solution. When our primary styles are not compatible, we can often find common ground by consciously negotiating from a secondary style.

All of us shift communication styles when speaking with different people in different contexts. For example, the default style of a man trying to pick up a woman for sex might be business, or "Let's make a deal." He may offer an expensive dinner and a night on the town in exchange for sex. If this same man were trying to get assistance in a car repair shop, his default communication style might be medical ("Let's find a cure.") or mechanical ("Let's figure out why this isn't working and how it can.").

The purpose of acknowledging our different styles and preferences in communication is not to categorize people or place limitations on them. It is to help us to become more able to focus on the issue itself and on meeting the needs of everyone involved.

Negotiating to Create Ecstatic Experiences

Now it's time to look at how to use language to create ecstatic events and relationships. Negotiation may seem like an odd word to use in an ecstatic or erotic context. But in fact, all negotiation really means is a discussion set up to produce an agreement. Whether the agreement you wish to reach is a multinational business deal or about the particulars of the hot date you and your partner are planning for this coming weekend, you'll need to have a discussion in order to reach an agreement. In an ecstatic context, negotiation is simply a form of mindfulness and conscious communication.

Negotiating can be done in a variety of styles and on virtually any topic. Whether the negotiation is to co-create an ecstatic experience or to solve a problem that has become an impediment to ecstasy, the basics of mindful and effective negotiation are the same. Here are some key steps:

Get the other person's perspective. What are their concerns? What do they need from you? What is their greatest need or desire in the eventual outcome?

Tell them what you need. Let the other person know what you need and why you need it. You may have different opinions about the best way to arrive at an ecstatic conclusion, but not about the overall ecstatic intention.

Think about some options beforehand. Many creative solutions are based on a joint modification of an idea that someone brings to the table. However, it's important not to become overly attached to your ideas. Anticipate why the other person might not agree with you and be prepared to offer alternatives.

Focus on solutions. Negotiation is not a debate. When we negotiate in order to solve a problem, our intention is to find a solution, not to place blame or be right. Don't try to prove the other person wrong. It's a waste of time and will only lead to an argument. If you find yourself overly attached to your point of view, ask yourself, "Would I rather be right, or would I rather be happy?" Keep your *attention* on the *intention*: to find a potentially ecstatic solution.

Negotiate at the right time. If either party is highly emotional, preoccupied with something else, stressed out, or exhausted, you are unlikely to reach any workable agreement.

Negotiate at the Resilient Edge of Resistance. Do not push someone beyond their emotional, physical, financial—or any other—resilient edge. Don't let yourself be pushed beyond your edge. Check in with each other. Take a break if you need to.

There are lots of reasons for keeping negotiations as fair and pleasant as possible, not the least of which is that at some future point, you may need to go back and renegotiate a portion of the agreement. Open relationships, for example, require constant renegotiation as circumstances, people, and desires change. Winning an ugly battle is never a win if no one wants to go back to the table to amend the agreement when things change.

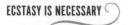

Negotiating for Ecstatic Relationships

Negotiating in our intimate relationships can be about a lot more than a search for solutions. It can be a wonderful opportunity to create "magic rooms" in which we can play out our deepest desires and dive into our Totality of Possibilities. In order to do that, the negotiation process must be a safe and fun space in which we may open up and express our deepest desires.

In intimate relationships the facts don't matter nearly as much as the feelings. If we're honest with ourselves, we'll admit that this is also true in business, politics, and international relations. Our society encourages us to focus on facts and debate, which it considers more "real" and more important than feelings. But even when we pretend that "it's all about the facts," our strongly held opinions are always accompanied by equally strong emotions. Famous negotiators have written books and taught expensive courses in which they encourage other negotiators not to show emotion. But that's not possible or effective in the realm of the erotic and the ecstatic. *Feelings are the essence of the ecstatic process.*

Negotiating in intimate relationships requires emotion-based guidelines:

Stay in touch with your deeper feelings and desires. In Chapter 1 you had the opportunity to discover your authentic needs and desires. Look over the notes in your journal, or do the exercise again prior to negotiating your next erotic adventure. (See page 42.)

Take responsibility for getting your needs met. Whether you are negotiating the plans for a date, or the future of a long-term erotic partnership, make sure you pay equal attention to your own needs and the needs of others. It's often most effective to focus on one person's needs at a time. If you are better at giving than receiving, set a timer so that all parties involved get equal time.

Stay at the Resilient Edge of Resistance of your feelings. Do not collapse into your emotions and allow the expression of your feelings to override the purpose of the negotiation, which is to find an agreement. Do not use your feelings as a controlling mechanism to make others feel guilty or sorry for you. Instead, breathe, stay present with your feelings, and allow your emotions to inform and guide you through the negotiation.

Communicate with an intention of self-discovery—not to produce a particular response from the other person. Imagine the person you are speaking with is interviewing you for a television show or a magazine article. This will focus your thinking and speaking. You'll likely find surprising new insights—about yourself, or about the issue you're discussing. When your intention in negotiation is self-discovery rather than convincing someone to see or do things your way, you'll avoid disappointment if they don't react the way you want them to. Plus, you are more likely to reach an agreement when the other person does not feel pushed to change in some way.

Focus on the future not the past. Talking about new erotic possibilities can bring up painful memories of disappointment, betrayal, shame, and guilt. Please remember that our brains have a tendency to believe that if something didn't work out well the first time it won't work out the next time. Breathe. Bring yourself back to the present moment. Look forward: How do you want the situation to look *now* and in the *future*?

See the big picture. Get some perspective. Imagine yourself looking down from a mountaintop. Realize how small your issue is in relation to all the issues of all the beings in your view. Or simply ask, "Who'll know in a hundred years?"

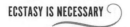

Open Heart Before Engaging Mouth

We've all heard the phrase "think before you speak." In our eager-ness—or desperation—to share our thoughts and feelings, our passion often gets the better of us and we say something that hurts someone else.

The need to express our feelings does not give us permission to turn off our brains. As Kahlil Gibran wrote,

> Your reason and your passion are the rudder and the sails of your seafaring soul. If either your sails or your rudder be broken, you can but toss and drift, or else be held at a standstill in mid-seas.

Although we want to be able to speak in plain, simple language, we also want to be thoughtful and gentle. How do we convey our message, especially when someone is resistant to hearing what we have to say? How do we talk about difficult subjects without losing control and saying things we later wish we hadn't?

Marshall B. Rosenberg, Ph.D., begins his book *Nonviolent Communication: A Language of Life* with:

> What I want in my life is compassion, a flow between myself and others based on a mutual giving from the heart.

Rosenberg, who developed the process called Nonviolent Communication, uses the term *nonviolence* the way Gandhi used it, "to refer to our natural state of compassion when violence has subsided from the heart." In some communities the same process is referred to as Compassionate Communication.

Compassionate Communication helps us reframe both how we express ourselves and how we hear others. It is a style of conscious communication rooted in our awareness of what we perceive, feel, or want. The basic model can be summarized this way:

When X happens . . . We describe X factually. We observe X without evaluating or making judgments about X.

. . . I feel Y . . . We distinguish our feelings from our thoughts. We especially try to access and express our deeper, softer, more subtle emotions.

. . . because I needed Z. We identify and speak about our fundamental needs and wants.

Would you be willing to . . . ? We request concrete actions that can be carried out in the present moment.

You don't need to speak according to this exact script. You simply need to be conscious of the four components: observations, feelings, needs, and requests.

For example, let's assume that your primary partner in your non-monogamous relationship has recently been seeing someone new and you are feeling some jealousy. To express this using Compassionate Communication, you might say, "When you are out with someone else and come home later than you said you would, I feel lost and alone because I'm afraid you won't come back to me. Could you please sit with me and tell me why you love me?"

The second part of Compassionate Communication is receiving empathetically—attempting to hear the need expressed by what the speaker just said. Your partner might reply, "Are you reacting to how many evenings I was out this week?" Or, "Are you feeling hurt because you would have liked more attention from me lately?" This kind of empathetic response allows you to express more of your feelings and ultimately get more of your needs met. In this case, you might not only receive what you requested—an outpouring of reasons why your partner loves you—but also a suggestion that the two of you go away for a romantic weekend.

One of the most effective ways to learn this model is to start with yourself. Much like the advice, "Put on your own oxygen mask before attempting to help others," we must learn to act compassionately toward ourselves before we can make a compassionate impact in our relationships and on the world.

Simply notice your next self-judgmental thought. For example: *How could I have forgotten to send Jane a birthday card? I am so stupid!* Ask yourself, *What need lies behind my judgment of myself as*

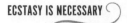
stupid? Perhaps the reason you forgot to send the card is because you have been working 60-hour weeks and need more unstructured time to yourself. How can you meet your own needs? Would you be willing to insist on a weekend off, even though it might mean upsetting your boss?

Compassionate Communication is a way of holding an intention of compassion for both ourselves and others. When we listen and treat ourselves with compassion we can more easily hold other higher intentions, such as pleasure, love, gratitude, and acceptance.

Active Listening

Active listening simply means conscious listening. It means that you are present to take in and appreciate someone else's message with relaxed, alive awareness.

We listen actively when we listen with the same level of conscious intention with which we speak. This is sometimes referred to as the "voice that listens." On a practical level, you may be listening for information, for something that will convince you, or excite you, or seduce you. But on a higher level, you could also listen with the intention to receive love, or with the intention to hear someone's true nature, or with the intention to experience someone's best. When you listen with your highest intentions, you'll find that you'll listen twice as long as you'll speak.

You can set a specific intention for your listening in advance of a conversation. For example, you might choose to listen with the intention to hear the expression of someone's most courageous self. Should the conversation become challenging, you can decide to listen with an appreciation of the bravery it takes for your beloved to speak about this sensitive issue. When you listen in this way, you release yourself from the expectations of a particular outcome and open yourself—and your partner—to the Totality of Possibilities of a bigger picture.

The first step in conscious listening is, of course, to be present.

You are present when you are actively receiving what is being said. You are not present if you are lost inside your own mind, planning your next speech. Mindful listening encourages an expanded awareness that also allows you to take in the nonverbal aspects of someone's language. Match your breath to their breath. Look into their eyes when you can—with the intention to see the best nature of their soul. Notice their body language. Does it seem tight and closed in? Open and expansive? Listen to the tone, speed, and pitch of their speech. Try to feel the emotion behind the language.

Stepping this wholly into someone's speech can feel scary, especially if the subject is difficult. Ironically though, when you are willing to totally commit to hearing someone, you can move past any uncomfortable stage quite quickly.

Feedback is another key piece of active listening. Some people think they are being gracious and respectful when they give you all the time in the world to speak and don't say a word or change facial expression until you ask them directly, "Well, how do you feel about this?" Silent, unresponsive listening—unless agreed upon in advance—can be unproductive and even destructive. Think about what happens in those stereotypical cartoons in which a psychoanalyst is sitting on a chair behind a patient who is lying on a couch facing away from them. The psychoanalyst begins the session with, "How are you today?" then proceeds to read a book for the rest of the hour while the patient runs the gamut from storytelling to intense emotional outbursts to profound realizations and only stops when the psychoanalyst says, "That's all for today. I'll see you next week." The patient gets off the couch and then thanks the psychoanalyst for their invaluable help.

Much like that patient, when we experience the void of silence we are tempted to fill it—with anything! If we are negotiating intense, troubled waters, desperately trying to make ourselves understood, we will tend to keep talking if we do not receive any feedback. We start to imagine what our partner might be thinking. We answer imaginary questions we think they must be silently asking. We may start expressing long-held feelings that have nothing to do with the topic at hand. We are likely to say things we don't really mean, or exaggerate our feelings just to get some re-action from our partner. The conversation can go completely off topic and out of control.

A conversation is not psychoanalysis. We need feedback. Al-though it is not appropriate to interrupt our partner, neither is it appropriate to sit in front of them impassive and silent. But let's suppose that you are the listener, and you are horrified, disap-pointed, saddened, or angry at what is being said. You really are speechless. Even if you cannot make a single constructive remark, you can acknowledge the speaker with a nod, or an, "I see."

One common and effective communication tool that is espe-cially helpful when you don't know what else to say, is to sum-marize what you believe the other person has said and repeat it back to them. For example, "I believe what I heard you say was that you feel I am not interested in the sexual pleasures available through bondage because I don't know enough about it. Did I get that right?"

"Yes, that's right."

Then the person can continue on with whatever they were saying, or you might say:

"Okay. May I ask a question?"

"Sure."

"Do you think I don't know enough about it because I don't have as much experience as you, or because I have not done enough research, or because I don't spend enough time thinking about it?"

Often, asking the right questions and getting clarification gives you a point of entry into the conversation that wasn't open to you while you were sitting silently with your horror, sadness, or disappointment.

If you are the speaker, stop talking once in a while—even if you have more to say—and check in with the other person. Ask, "Do you have anything you'd like to say?" Or, "I'm curious to hear how you feel about what I just said." Or, "Was I clear on that last point? Do you want to tell me what you heard?"

There are times when someone may need or want to talk without interruption. This can provide an opportunity for the speaker to access their deeper feelings and may lead to insights that would not have been revealed another way. This style of speaking—sometimes referred to as a talking circle—is also good for group discussions and brainstorming sessions. The rules for a talking circle are simple: Each person is allowed to speak until they feel they have said everything they need to say. Then it's the next person's turn to speak. Depending on the nature of the circle, this next person may speak about their feelings, or may reply to the person who has just spoken.

There is one modification I will sometimes add to a talking-circle format to more fully support someone in saying everything they need to say. When someone says they are finished, I sometimes ask, "Is there more?" This question often prompts the realization of some hidden insight—and in the case of someone trying to express their erotic desire—the most exciting sexual scenario. Remember, the question is, "Is there more?" *Never* ask someone, "Are you done?" That's a sure way of shutting down any possibility of a further creative thought or a deeper emotion.

Watch for Unspoken Expectations

Be careful that you aren't basing your agreements on unspoken conditions, expectations, or assumptions.

When my friend Kevin broke up with his longtime girlfriend, Laura, they agreed that they would alternate their attendance at a holiday festival they used to attend together. Shortly after their breakup, Kevin went to the festival alone and had a wonderful time. Upon his return, Laura asked Kevin for a period of non-communication while she healed from the break up. Kevin was sad about this and feared that they would no longer be friends. In my conversation with him about the festival and their arrangement, he said, "We made an agreement that I would go this year but not go next year, so that she could go alone or with someone else. But now I'm reconsidering that agreement." "Why?" I asked. "Because," he said, "when we made that agreement it was based on the fact that we would remain friends."

"Oh really?" I asked. "Did you state that condition when you made the agreement?"

"Well no, not exactly. But I just assumed that's the way it would work out."

"So friendship is a condition that you are now applying retroactively and unilaterally to your agreement with Laura? Kevin, friendship was never mentioned or agreed upon as a condition. It was something you *assumed*."

In short, if a condition is not clearly stated in the original agreement, you cannot expect anyone to live up to it. However, we all make unconscious assumptions based upon our own values, needs, and culturally imposed beliefs. We assume that other people— especially those closest to us—share our values, needs, and beliefs. We are often not aware that we have made an assumption until someone's behavior runs contrary to our expectations. When that happens, we either need to honor our original agreement, or ask to renegotiate the agreement, admitting our unconscious assumption.

Ecstatic Communication

Have you ever stayed up all night reveling in the bliss of a magical conversation with that special someone with whom you have recently fallen deeply in love? If so, you've had a direct experience of how communication itself can be an ecstatic experience. The process of negotiating sensual and sexual adventures can also be delightful. In the preceding chapters, we have explored our values, needs, and desires. We discovered what we needed in order to feel safe. We established our boundaries and learned how to take an erotic risk. Now we also know how to compassionately communicate all of these things to someone else. Our last step is to make this communication passionate, playful, and fun.

Communication as an ecstatic experience in and of itself is

both an exquisite experience and a powerful intention. Too often, in our search for ecstasy, we unconsciously assume that our usual habits, conventions, and customs will lead us where we'd like to go. We may take for granted that our partner wants what we want, and that things will go as we wish. Consciously and deliberately writing down our desires can feel a little awkward at first. Once you try it, however, you may discover that it can be an intensely delightful turn-on.

EXERCISE: YES NO MAYBE LIST

Take a large piece of paper and make a list of all the erotic, sexual, kinky activities you can think of, including those that you are not personally interested in. If possible, do this with a lover, a friend, or in a group. Other people will come up with activities that you haven't thought of. As an added benefit, any time we talk about sex in a playful and positive manner with one or more other people, we reduce shame and give people permission to be more erotically adventurous.

Once you have your large list, take another piece of paper and divide it into three columns titled *Yes*, *No*, and *Maybe*. Write all the items that you like or that you would like to try in the *Yes* column. In the *No* column, write all the things that you have absolutely no interest in at this time. In the *Maybe* column, write all the things you might like to try if you felt safe enough, and if all the circumstances were right.

The next time you want to plan an erotic encounter—which, after you've made this list could be immediately—go back over your Yes/No/Maybe list. Choose from the *Yes* column all the activities that you want and need in your erotic encounter right now—for example—oral sex, a spanking, and an orgasm. Then select some items from the *Maybe* list—perhaps an erotic food fight, biting and scratching, or hair pulling. If the person you are

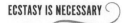

negotiating with is happy to give you oral sex, a spanking, and an orgasm, and is also potentially interested in an erotic food fight, biting and scratching, or hair pulling, you're with the right partner on the right night. If this person is not interested in giving you oral sex, a spanking, and an orgasm, you might want to find someone else to play with. Or, you could revisit your list to see if other activities would fulfill the same desires and needs. Or you might wait until another night when this person is able to give you what you want.

Even negotiations about potentially uncomfortable subjects such as safer sex can be made passionate, playful, and fun. (Those of you who have already established safer-sex protocols with your current partner(s) can skip ahead to page 203. You can always come back to this when you need it.) I suggest you prepare in advance for this conversation with a little two to three minute personal statement of your sexual health status and safer-sex practices. You can use it in the consent/negotiation/sharing process with any new partner before any sexual activity takes place. Here's an example:

> **Hi. My name is** _____. **I have tested positive for** _____[insert name of sexually transmitted infection, if any. Give details if appropriate.]. **I was last tested** _____ [insert how long ago] **for** _____ [insert name(s) of other STIs and give result of those tests]. **My safer-sex practices are** __ _____. [insert how you practice safer sex, for example, "I use condoms for all penetrative sex, including oral. I use plastic wrap for oral sex on women. I use gloves for penetrative sex with my hands. I use condoms and gloves on all sex toys."] **I love** _____ [insert types of sexual activity you enjoy or would be interested in doing with this person.]. **I am not fond of** _____[insert types of sexual activity you do not enjoy or do not want to do with this person.].

In order to make this little elevator speech a turn-on instead of a turnoff, give the details of any sexually transmitted infections simply and succinctly. Slow down and take a bit more time to describe your safer-sex practices. Show your enthusiasm when you tell them the types of sexual activity you like. Then, ask them their status and safer-sex practices. Listen passionately and without judgment. When you are both finished, you can begin negotiations about how and if you might want to play together.

Thus far, our discussion of ecstatic communication has focused on the written or spoken word. Here are four sensual exercises designed to explore and expand your nonverbal ecstatic communication skills.

Exercise: A Sensuous Buffet

In this exercise, you'll feed your blindfolded partner morsels of a variety of foods. Your partner will nonverbally communicate their delight—or disgust—with each taste.

   Each of you will begin by gathering as wide a variety of tastes as possible. Be sure to include sweet, sour, bitter, and salty tastes, as well as a variety of textures. Here are a few ideas: chocolate, fruit, mustard, whipped cream, salsa, a sparkling beverage, a salty snack, diluted lemon juice, sweet or sour pickles.

   Giving partner: Blindfold your partner. (Or for extra fun, put them in bondage.) Just make sure that the only sense completely blocked out for the entire exercise is sight. Now, feed your partner. Go s-l-o-w-l-y. Run a tasty morsel over their lips and tongue but don't let them bite it. Allow them to experience the aroma, texture, and temperature of the food, and only then let them have a small bite. Feed your partner with the intention of helping them appreciate every nuance of the food.

   Receiving partner: Enter as totally as you can into the experience of the food and of being fed. If you like the morsel you taste, ask for more by making "yum" sounds, by reaching for more with your tongue, or by licking your partner's fingers. Express your displeasure by scrunching up your face, making "icklike" noises, or turning away.

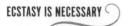

After a certain number of tastes, or a certain amount of time, switch places.

This exercise can get ridiculously funny. It can also cause you to drop deliciously deeply into your body, your connection with each other, and into the flavors of the food.

EXERCISE: BODY PAINTING

In this exercise you'll communicate with your partner by means of color and touch.

You can buy non-toxic body paints in sex shops, novelty shops, and art supply stores. A quick Internet search will turn up many outlets. You can use your hands, paintbrushes, or sponges to apply the paint. You need no artistic skill. Simply invite your nude partner to lie down on a paint-friendly surface (an old sheet placed over a plastic drop cloth works well) and declare your love, lust, and/or delight for this beautiful being by covering them with color. You can turn them into an abstract expressionist painting or a creature from the woods. You can paint them to express how you see them, or to bring out some aspect of their inner beauty.

This exercise is a tactile experience as well as a visual one, so be sure that each stroke of color feels as good as it looks.

Receiving partner: While you're being painted, show your appreciation for the sensual touch with moans and groans. If the brushes tickle, squeal in protest—or delight! When you see yourself as a completed work of art, act out whatever or whoever you have become.

EXERCISE: A SHARED SHOWER

In this exercise you'll communicate with your lover with scent, texture, touch, water—and fruit! Before inviting your beloved into the shower for a wordless bathing ritual, gather luxurious scents and textures. In addition to washcloths, loofah sponges, and bath salts, you can slice oranges, grapefruit, limes, and lemons in halves or quarters and use them as bath sponges. Rub them all over your lover's body. The aroma of the citrus is amplified by the hot water and steam.

Show your lover how much you adore their body by how you touch and how long you linger. You can drip the fruit juice into your lover's mouth or lick it off their body. Show your appreciation with moans, groans, kisses, licks, and bites. You can bathe each other simultaneously, or take turns giving and receiving.

EXERCISE: BREATHING AND EYE-GAZING

This exercise is simple, but not always easy, especially if it's new for you. Breathing and eye-gazing are deeply intimate acts and it can take a few minutes to get past the awkward, giggly stage.

Sit comfortably across from your partner and gently gaze into their eyes. Feel free to choose just one eye if that makes it easier to keep your gaze consistent.

Now breathe. Take full, gentle breaths. Allow your breath to synchronize with your partner's.

There is no need to do anything more. Just breathe together and gaze into your partner's eyes.

Sometimes you can feel an emotional conversation taking place. Other times it seems that nothing—and everything—is being said all at once. Sometimes your partner's face will seem to change.

When you are finished, close your eyes and meditate for a few moments. Silently witness your feelings.

Whether the language you use in the creation of—or in the midst of—an ecstatic encounter is verbal or nonverbal, the emphasis is on love—sharing love, co-creating love, returning to love. When your intention is to speak from a space of love—for yourself as well as the person you are speaking with—the words are merely a jumping-off point. You become the meaning of the words. When communication itself crosses over into the ecstatic, it feels more like you are drinking in your partner than listening to them. The silence between the words becomes intoxicating— more significant than the words themselves. The meaning shines through your eyes, your touch, your very being.

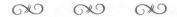

CHAPTER 7

Living an Ecstatic Life

In the preceding pages, we have looked at many of the ways in which we lose touch with our ecstatic selves, and we have practiced techniques to bring ourselves back into alignment. You may have already discovered that it's easier than you thought to create a single ecstatic experience. It can, however, be more challenging to create ecstatic experiences on a regular basis—or to stitch those ecstatic experiences together into the fabric of an ecstatic life.

Achieving an ecstatic life is more possible than you might imagine. My concept of an ecstatic life does not demand that I walk around in a constant state of bliss. That would be nice, of course, but I don't want to live under the pressure of that expectation. I need to imagine a level of ecstasy that I know I could possibly achieve. Therefore, my concept of an ecstatic life means that I have the ability to access ecstatic moments when I want them, and that I am able to allow more and more of the moments of my life to be ecstatic. Even when things are difficult, painful, and upsetting, I know that I will ultimately be able to use the elements of whatever is happening to create an ecstatic experience, if not now, then in the reasonably near future. For me, living an ecstatic life means looking upon ecstasy as my spiritual practice.

Living an ecstatic life is an evolutionary process. It's not like going to a spa for a weekend of pampering—it's more like meditation. An ecstatic life requires commitment. If you've ever begun a meditation practice, you know it's slow going at first. You may only be in an actual meditative state 2 percent of the time. You spend the rest of your time adjusting your posture, your breath, and watching your thoughts. When you finally relax your body and your mind, it's as if a magic door appears and you step into a meditative universe. My personal image for an ecstatic practice is surfing. I know the waves are always out there waiting for me— somewhere. I need the discipline to discover where they are on any given day, and then show up prepared. I must have the patience to sit on my surfboard until I sense the right wave forming, and then line up my board in the perfect position to catch the wave. Once I do, a combination of experience, exhilaration, and skill keeps me flying all the way in to shore.

In the introduction of this book I talked about The Something More Factor—that innate knowledge we all have that there is something more out there waiting for us if only we could find it. Even if the only action you have taken in support of your ecstatic future is to read this book, that's an important step into your Something More. You now know why you do sex—that is, *if* you do sex and if you *want* to do sex. You have some deeper awareness of your values, needs, and desires. You know how to create a personal safety net, as well as how to set limits and boundaries. You've learned the building blocks of sexual self-esteem and courage, and you have greater insight into the kinds of communication that are most likely to help you get your needs and desires met. Finally, you have learned to give yourself permission to experience your ecstasy and you know that you can sit in an easy relationship with any guilt or shame that arises. Perhaps along the way you've also had a glimpse of your Something More. In this chapter you're going to learn how to live more of your life in the ecstatic and ongoing revelation of that Something More.

In BDSM there is a category called edge play. Edge play, as the words imply, means any activity that rides along the razor's edge of someone's limits. These limits might be physical, emotional, or mental. An edge-play scene might challenge someone's limits of fear, intense sensation, or even their ability to receive unconditional love. Much in the same way that a great athlete sets a goal to break a record or achieve a personal best, the ecstatic explorer sets their intention, then carefully and intensely trains their body, mind, and spirit to meet that challenge.

In ecstatic terms, no matter which activities we prefer—sex, trance dancing, sports, or branding—we will eventually come to the end of safe and familiar territory. When we reach that point, we can either turn around and go back to the familiar, or leap off the ledge into our Totality of Possibilities. When you have begun to treat ecstasy as a meditative practice, you come to understand that leaping off the ledge is not only the most fun option, in a paradoxical way, it's also the safest. Turning around and giving up—going back to being who we were before we ever glimpsed this edge and its possibilities—is not only disappointing, it's also unhealthy. We are meant to challenge ourselves and grow. We seek ecstatic expression the way flowers seek the sun. We do not bloom in the shade of our regrets or past accomplishments.

The specifics of each individual's ecstatic path are different, but ecstatic practice produces some common experiences. When I am on my ecstatic path, I feel like I'm living my life on purpose—consciously and with intention. I am living in alignment with my values and my life's mission. I feel authentic, natural, and even ordinary. It often takes a remark by somebody else to remind me how extraordinary my life really is. As my teaching partner, Chester, once said as we were loading up the car to drive to a weekend erotic massage workshop, "Ho hum, yet another weekend of naked people breathing, moaning, and writhing around in pleasure—just another day at the office!" When I'm living my ecstatic life, I am in awe of all the places my work and my life take me. I also feel like it is all completely normal.

The ecstatic path is borderless and boundary-less. Whether I experience this in the afterglow of an orgasm, during meditation, or simply while walking down the street on a beautiful day, the feeling is the same—there is no separation between me and everything else. Paradoxically, I feel both connected to everyone and everything else, and also completely free. I am not bound by anyone's opinions, ideologies, or demands.

An essential and inevitable quality of an ecstatic life is humor. Let's face it, sex is funny. Just like most experiences that demand you lose yourself totally in the present moment, the longer you explore sex the sillier it can seem. This is a very good thing. Gigglegasms are one of life's most powerful and exquisite pleasures. I enjoy them so much that I don't even mind if the joke is on me.

One of the ways I measure how closely I am following my ecstatic path is by observing the level of regret I do, or do not, feel. I certainly have had my share of disappointments, pain, and betrayals, and yet I don't regret those experiences. I also can't think of anything significant in my life that I regret not having done. Yes, there are some things I might have done differently, but even the things that did not work out the way I wished have led to some other experience rich with ecstasy or ecstatic potential. So instead of regrets, I have goals. Despite the fact that my personal image for an ecstatic life is surfing, the truth is, I still have not learned how to surf properly. I have played around with surfboards, but I have not yet successfully stood up on a board and ridden it into the shore. One of my goals and my promises to myself is to take surfing lessons in warm tropical waters. For me, the key to not having any regrets is to keep these promises to myself that will fulfill my deepest desires.

Finally, an ecstatic life is life lived in amazement. I am consistently amazed at life in all its weird and wacky permutations. I am amazed by how much I've learned over the years. I'm equally amazed by how little I know.

What would/does an ecstatic life feel like for you?

Keys to An Ecstatic Life

Today I was asked the question; How would a life of ecstasy look
for me? My answer? To walk with a sparkle in my eyes, a tingle
in my balls, and shining from my heart.

— Danniel, Urban Tantra® Professional Training Program graduate

While mapping out this chapter, I was facilitating my Urban Tantra
Professional Training Program in Australia. My training program
is designed to help people who work in any capacity in the field of
sexuality to create, maintain, and expand their careers by practicing and teaching conscious sexuality, using techniques borrowed
from a variety of sacred sex practices.

The Australian training program was especially large, varied,
and passionate. We spent an entire week exploring expanded, ecstatic states, and learning how to teach others to do the same. The
old adage that we all teach what we most need to learn held true
for most of us. We were experts in our knowledge of how to live an
ecstatic life, and equally expert in forgetting to do it for ourselves.

So for the closing circle of our week together I asked the group
what three things they were each going to promise to do for themselves to make their life more ecstatic. The resulting conversation
informs the rest of this chapter. The answers to the question I
posed demonstrated that not only is ecstatic living a regular practice, but that there are also ways to approach the practice that
make it easier, more effective, and more fun.

Let's begin by looking at the aspects of your life that hold the greatest potential for ecstasy. If your life seems lacking in ecstatic potential at the moment, ask yourself, "Which areas of my life do I *wish* were more ecstatic?" Sex? Relationships? Work? Children? If an ecstatic life feels a long way off—as though the thought of creating even one ecstatic moment would be a challenge—start small. Pick one area of your life and focus there. Ecstasy is contagious. Not only does it spread from person to person, it eventually infects all areas of your life.

The approach to an ecstatic life is similar to the approaches we've explored for ecstatic experiences and relationships. We've already discussed some of these points, but it's worth revisiting them in this broader context.

Become lovers with your evolving self. In Chapter 2, you spent a considerable amount of time getting to know who you were as an authentic erotic and ecstatic being. The exercises in that chapter and in Chapter 3 reacquainted you with both your past and present selves. You are, however, not limited to the past and the present. You are also in relationship with your *evolving* self—the you who is creating your future. Your evolving self exists in this present moment. In order to step forward into your Something More you need to be in a consistent, friendly relationship with your evolving self. This relationship might feel scary. You may not be sure who this new person is, or how well you really want to know them. You may be afraid that they will lead you down some dangerous path. Avoiding your evolving self will not save you from your future. It *will* prevent you from playing a role in the conscious creation of your future. Walking with awareness of the presence of your evolving self will help you recognize the next doors that will open for you.

Radically accept—everything. Radical Acceptance is the practice of accepting things as they are with no expectation of change. When we accept things the way they are and are willing to be happy and satisfied with that, almost any situation can be turned into an experience that—if not ecstatic in itself—can lead to a place of peace and no regrets, both of which contribute to an ecstatic life. Remember, Radical Acceptance provides the opportunity for finding infinitely more creative and ecstatic possibilities, and it paves the way for positive change.

Live what you love. This is hardly a new maxim, but it's essential to an ecstatic life. Do as much of what you love as you possibly can. Do as little as you must of anything you don't like. The more you commit to what you love, the easier it is to let the rest be handled by someone else who enjoys it more. Pay attention to your intuitive energy meter. Remember to ask yourself: "Do I feel an energy gain or an energy drain in this situation, or around this person?" Eliminate or minimize your exposure to anything or anyone that drains your energy. Embrace that which feeds you.

Whatever you're doing—do it wholeheartedly. Do not hold back. Give yourself over completely. Be bigger than you think you are. Be more than you've ever been. Be too much.

Embrace and celebrate your inner teenager. What was your passion at age 13? Or age 16? How did you pursue that passion? What was your most compelling reason for pursuing this passion? How did you behave if people told you that your passion was wrong, silly, or a waste of time? Revisit your most ecstatic, stubborn, passionate, activist years. Take notes. See your inner teenager as a vital part of your authentic adult self.

On a related note, **redefine aging**. What if as we got older we became more passionate instead of less? What if life were more fun? What if age freed us from the fear of others' judgments? What if we became more hopeful and less jaded? What might we accomplish—for ourselves and others—if we combined the wisdom of our years with the passion of our youth?

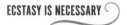

Go to the edge. Fall off. See what's there. Start a love affair with your own fear. Imagine your fear as your best friend. Throw a fear party. Invite all your friends and all their fears. Dance with all your emotions.

Seize the moment—and stay in it. Slow down! Spend as much time in each present moment as you can. We often complain that we want more time in our lives. Why would the universe give us *more* time if we can't appreciate the time we *do* have? Stretch each present moment to its fullest. See how much ecstasy you can savor in each moment of the day.

Beginning A Daily Ecstatic Practice

Ecstasy is an embodied holistic practice. You cannot simply think your way into a more ecstatic experience or life. Certainly, how you think and what you think about is critical. But it's not the whole picture. My breath and energy orgasm—which the Discovery Channel producers at first referred to as "thinking off"—was brought about by a lot more than just thinking. It involved physical, emotional, and spiritual practices. As I mentioned earlier, some people can reach orgasm simply by using their imagination. Most of us can't. Yet, almost anyone can learn a breath and energy orgasm technique in which imagination is combined with physical techniques. It's just the same with ecstasy.

The difference between ecstatic states and states of pleasure, happiness, or comfort is that ecstatic experiences embrace the entire being: physical, social, emotional, and spiritual. Creating an embodied ecstatic practice is similar to establishing a meditation practice, or an exercise routine—you have to love it, or at least be able to learn to love it—or you won't do it for long. You also have to stick to it long enough for it to become a habit—until it becomes something that you'll miss if you stop. If you have ever started some new or expanded erotic practice—either alone or with a partner—and weren't able to maintain it, either you probably didn't give it long enough to allow it to become habitual, or you weren't significantly turned on by your choice.

One of the most common sexual complaints is a lack of desire. We are conditioned to believe that desire is something that we must feel before we can be sexual. If we are not turned on prior to making love, there must be something wrong with us, our relationship, or the way we feel about our partner. Anemia, diabetes or another major disease, alcohol or drug abuse, certain prescription drugs, and hormonal imbalances can all adversely affect desire. And certainly, if you are in an abusive or otherwise unhealthy relationship, you may not want to have sex with your partner. But in a large percentage of cases, lack of sexual desire is caused by lack of sex.

Sexual desire resembles meditation or exercise, in that the more you do it, the more you want to do it. Like any habit, the more sex you have, the more sex you're likely to want. The less sex you have—with yourself or with someone else—the less likely you are to think about sex or feel the desire to do it. Most people do not have physical impediments to desire. They are simply out of the habit of desiring. This is why establishing a regular ecstatic physical practice—sexual as well as nonsexual—is so beneficial.

The following suggestions will help you create your own ecstatic practice. We'll start with physical practices, then fold in social, emotional, and spiritual elements.

Ecstatic Physical Practices

Engaging in ecstatic and erotic physical pursuits seems so obviously pleasurable that you'd think we'd all be doing it on a regular basis. But we're not. The demands of everyday life often supersede our need and desire for physical and sexual pleasure. And we are often hesitant to start a new practice for fear that—once again—we won't follow through. You do not need to do every single one of the practices that follow. Start with one or two—the ones that appeal to you most—and practice them regularly. As you progress, you can expand or modify your practice with new choices.

Start your day with an embodied ecstatic practice. What's the first thought you think when you wake up in the morning? Do you immediately think, *This is going to be the best day* ever. *I can hardly wait to jump in to all the possible delights that this day has in store for me!* Or do you think about all the unpleasant things you'll have to do, all the problems you'll face, and all of yesterday's unfinished messes that you'll have to clean up?

Start your day with both a positive thought and with medibation—the practice of conscious masturbation followed by meditation. Practice simple sex magic before you begin to raise sexual energy. Envision a delightful day in front of you. When you have your day imagined as perfectly as you can, begin to masturbate, dedicating your erotic energy to your vision. Then simply let go of your vision—release it to the universe. Now pleasure yourself to orgasm. Think of your medibation as orgasmic prayer.

Of course, you could also begin your day with a positive thought and any other physical practice you find ecstatic. (Go back to Chapter 1 if you need inspiration.) But if you are avoiding medibation simply because you have gotten out of the habit of sex, I strongly suggest you consider a specifically sexual morning practice.

Use the techniques of expanded orgasmic states to bring ecstasy into your daily life. You can use the same simple techniques that I use to have a breath and energy orgasm to make any activity more ecstatic. If you'd like to incorporate them into a full breath and energy orgasm, see Afterglow D for complete instructions.

- *Breathe.* Become breath positive. Take big, full breaths—exhale with an audible sigh. Set the alarm on your mobile phone to ring every hour. When the alarm goes off take ten big, full breaths—no matter where you are. Be a public example of the ecstatic power of breath.

  Learning and practicing a variety of breath techniques will open the door to a Totality of Possibilities of ecstatic experiences. Take a pranayama yoga class. Learn breath and energy orgasms (See Afterglow D). Attend a Holotropic Breathwork™ workshop. Holotropic Breathwork™ combines accelerated breathing with evocative music to allow people to access non-ordinary states of consciousness. It is—I can state from experience—better than psychedelic drugs.

Become addicted to your own breath.

- *Make sounds.* One surefire way to have bigger, better, more intense orgasms is to open up your throat and make some noise. However, many of us are hesitant about making noise during sex. I believe that this is in large part due to the Quiet-and-Quick Rule we learned in adolescence. When we were first exploring our sexuality through masturbation, we needed to be quiet to avoid being discovered, and we had to be quick so that we could be assured of an orgasm before someone knocked on our door. The most reliable way to accomplish both of these goals was to hold our breath. In doing so, we established two habits guaranteed to limit our sexual and ecstatic pleasure: holding our breath and not making sounds. You can begin to change these habits. Start vocalizing as you raise sexual energy. You do not have to scream (although you can if you like—just throw a pillow over your mouth if you live in an apartment with thin walls) and you do not have to speak words. Just open your throat and make some sounds.

- *Exercise your PC muscle.* First, find your PC (pubococcygeus) muscle. Imagine you are in the bathroom peeing and someone unexpectedly opens the bathroom door. What do you do? You stop peeing. Feel that? That little muscle that stopped the flow of urine? That's your PC muscle. PC squeezes (sometimes called Kegels) exercise the pelvic floor muscles that people of all genders need

217

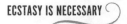

for robust sexual health and vitality. Not only that, PC squeezes act as erotic energy pumps, moving your sexual energy up from your genitals up into the rest of your body.

You can do your PC squeezes anywhere: standing in line at the ATM, waiting for a traffic light to change, walking down the street, or working out at the gym. They'll also keep you from nodding off in boring business meetings and classes.

- *Shake your booty!* Your pelvis is your sexual power center. You need a strong, loose pelvis to thrust, undulate, and swing your hips forward (or backward) to meet a lover's thrust, as well as to move sexual energy throughout your body.

  Begin by swinging your hips in a circle to the right eight times. Now circle to the left eight times. Now, pretend you are a belly dancer and move your hips in a figure eight: right, center, left, center. Let it be sexy! Throw is some PC squeezes for extra juiciness.

Connect to your orgasmic energy. Give yourself permission to be orgasmic. If you are genitally non-orgasmic for some reason, research ways that you can achieve another form of orgasm. Remember, if you are alive, you have orgasmic and ecstatic potential. Quadriplegics with no feeling below the neck have had orgasms when a one-inch square patch of skin on their neck was stimulated just right. There is always a path to ecstasy. Self-pleasure instead of self-medicating with food, alcohol, drugs, television, or the Internet. Prioritize this essential part of self-care.

Expand your sexuality. Whether or not you have a partner, commit to being more sensual and sexual. Broaden your definition of sex to include more activities and experiences. Try something new—a new position, or toy, or activity. Re-examine your sexual boundaries with the intention of seeing if you'd like to relax some of them. Think of sex as adult play, and set up a play date.

Take yourself on a weekly date. That's right; this date is just between you and you. On your date explore a new pleasure or fulfill a new desire. You might take yourself to a sex shop to pick out a new toy and a hot video. Or you might learn how to have a breath and energy orgasm. Or perhaps there is a sexy lecture or workshop nearby. If you long for a companion, imagine you're dating your inner teenager, or your evolving self. Let them choose the activity for your date.

Dance your sexy dance. Many of us have an uneasy relationship with dance and dancing. Perhaps you were ridiculed in a high school phys ed dance class, or you hold painful memories of school dances where you felt awkward, unattractive, and clumsy. Reclaim your body's natural desire to dance. Put on some music with a strong beat and move! If this makes you feel self-conscious or silly, wear a blindfold. If you live in a small space and fear that you'll crash into things, simply plant your feet and shake or dance in place. Do not worry about what you look like, even if you are by yourself. Dance any way you feel and let your entire body move as it wishes for at least 15 minutes. Enjoy the sensations of dancing. You might even feel like an invisible, nameless partner is dancing you around the room.

Handle nagging physical problems. Do you have a persistent physical issue that you have been meaning to deal with but just haven't gotten around to yet? Remember our discussion of energy gain versus energy drain? The physical problem you're avoiding is draining energy that you could be using for ecstatic expression. Whether it's poor eyesight, back pain, sexual pain, or any other chronic condition, practice self-love and self-care by getting support.

Dissolve the boundary between your body and nature. Whether you live in a big city, a small town, or in the country, take a moment each day to establish a connection to a natural element. This could be as simple as taking a walk in which you lose yourself in the

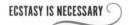

feeling of the sun on your skin, or feel yourself absorbed into the blue of the sky. You could hug a tree, listen intently to the song of a bird, or even spend quality time with your dog. A key aspect of ecstatic experience is connection to all that is. Consciously practicing this connection on a daily basis keeps that ecstatic channel open.

Receive full-body touch. Whether you pay for it or exchange it with a friend or lover, get touched! When a massage or lovemaking is not available, enjoy full-body hugs.

Ecstatic Social Practices

Increasing numbers of us are self-employed, freelancing, and/or working from home. This means that more and more of us are working alone. These solo and self-directed work-styles frequently involve working longer hours with fewer days off. Almost all of the people in my Australian professional training program fit into one of these solo work-style categories, and not surprisingly, the most popular answer to the question "What would make your life more erotic and ecstatic?" was to spend more quality time with like-minded folks.

Ecstatic beings are not islands. It is certainly possible to have an ecstatic experience by yourself, but it is usually a lot easier and more fun if other people are involved. In order to live an ecstatic *life*, connections with other people are vital.

When we are immersed in our busy, overworked lives, time spent with anyone other than our primary partner—if we have one—can seem like a luxury. It can seem impossible to coordinate schedules with the people we would really like to see, or to find the time to make new friends. Plus, we may be so out of the habit of socializing, we don't even know where to begin. Start by setting aside two hours, or one evening a week. Contact good friends you haven't seen or spoken to in a while. Find one who is available when you are. If they live too far away to meet in person, set up a phone or video Skype date.

Cultivate new relationships. *What?!* you may be thinking. *I don't have time for the ones I have now!* Relax. Using your two hours or one evening a week to meet new people does not obligate you to spend some prescribed amount of time with them in the future. First, ask yourself, "What's my priority? Where have I been feeling a gap in my social life?" Is it making new friends? Finding sex partners? Dating in hopes of creating a relationship? Professional support? Creative inspiration? Head in the direction of your most pressing need or desire.

One client of mine, Trish, was desperate to meet a lover with whom to practice Tantra. She lived in a very small town and she could not seem to find anyone suitable in her area. In our first session, I asked her whether she was willing to move. She gave me a long list of reasons why moving did not feel sensible, practical, or possible right now. So, I helped her create a wish list describing her ideal lover, then guided her toward Internet dating sites geared to people interested in a sexual/spiritual connection. Nothing seemed to work. No one she met online lived anywhere near her. Finally, she turned on me in frustration, "Nothing is working! What is wrong with you? Why can't you help me?" I said, "I can help you, but I don't think you'll like it." "Of course I want you to help me. This is *so* important to me," she pleaded. "Okay, I said. "If you are that sincerely committed to meeting someone, you're either going to have to be willing to travel a lot, or move." Trish remained unwilling to relocate, and initially had another long list of reasons why she could not travel to events where she was likely to meet someone who might be willing to travel to see her, either occasionally or regularly. However, over the course of the next few months, Trish was able to find both the time and the money to travel to a weekend event where she did, indeed, meet a potential partner.

If you live in an area where the right ecstatic companions are difficult or impossible to find, you may need to travel or relocate in order to meet collaborators with whom to build your dreams.

Avoid social obligations. Pursue social opportunities. The rare social obligation—even if it's deadly dull—will not prevent you from living an ecstatic life. But if you allow yourself to be lured into too many of these so-called obligatory functions, you'll find yourself being drained of the time and energy you would otherwise have to devote to more meaningful interactions.

A social obligation does not have to be an energy drain. Often it can be converted into a social opportunity. For example, if you feel drained by the obligation to attend a banquet honoring your boss, you could convert it into an opportunity by inviting that funny, charming friend you don't see very often to be your date.

If you can't imagine a way to convert a social obligation into a social opportunity, ask yourself, how much of an obligation is it anyway? To whom are you obligated? What will be lost if you don't go? I have made my distaste of weddings so clear to everyone I know that no one who knows me well would even think of inviting me to one. Of course, there are certain social obligations—particularly involving family members—that you may feel you cannot avoid. There would be just too high a price to pay for your refusal to participate. If that's the case, go, make the best of it, and then balance it out by pursuing a social *opportunity* within the next week.

A social opportunity can be found anywhere and anytime you have a high probability of meeting delightful people who share one or more of your passions. It could be an erotic massage workshop, an evening of trance dancing, a gourmet dessert-baking evening, or a birthday celebration at a spa. Try and arrange at least two social opportunities for every social obligation. If you need inspiration and assistance finding opportunities, search the Internet for meet-up groups in your area. There are meet-up groups for virtually every interest.

Create an Ecstasy Lab. Do you have a place where you can explore sex—or any other ecstatic pursuit—consciously, with people you like and respect? The concept of an Ecstasy Lab was created by my Australian colleague, Avika de Vine, who wanted to find a way to explore specific erotic pleasures with other conscious explorers in an environment that is both social and educational. Whether you call your event a salon, a gathering, a playshop, or a lab, the intention is to create a "magic room" to explore sex that is more organized than a party, but less formal than a workshop. Meetings can be organized around a theme, an activity, or a speaker. There may be less than a dozen members, or it may grow to include over 100.

If you're interested in starting an Ecstasy Lab, begin by writing a mission statement. A mission statement is simply a written intention for your group. Craft your intention so that it involves and benefits all members of the group you wish to create. For example, "My intention is to bring together people with a wide variety of sexual talents and preferences for a monthly exploration of the sacred eroticism common to us all." Your intention should be able to be stated in a sentence or two. Keep it simple. A written mission statement will help you stay focused on the purpose of your group and help you make the correct decisions about appropriate activities, venues, and members.

Allow your relationships to change. Once you have made a commitment to nurture more frequent and more numerous ecstatic and erotic relationships, you may find that you are spending more time with your new friends and less time with others. This may worry you—or your old friends. Consider this: There is no possible way you could maintain all your relationships—at the same intensity as they originally existed—for your entire life. Remember your best friend in grade school with whom you spent hours playing? Or your best friend in high school with whom you spent even more hours on the phone? How about all the other best friends and lovers you have had? There is no possible way you could sustain all these relationships simultaneously. Love may be unlimited, but time is not.

Not only does the cast of characters change in the epic movie that is your life, but your relationship with each of those characters changes even as you are engaging in the relationship. One of

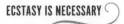

the most impossible—and dangerous—intentions to hold is, "This is perfect. I never want it to change. I want us to be just like this forever."

> We tend to think of relationships as static, as if we could just get into them, assume a position inside them and then continue to hold it, essentially without changing forever, world without end. But in fact our relationships are fluid, vivid, mercurial, and constantly changing.
>
> — Daphne Rose Kingma, *The Future of Love*

Relationships are *supposed* to change. It's the nature of relationship. It's what makes them living, breathing entities. Throughout this book, we have been reminded that ecstatic experience happens at the Resilient Edge of Safety and Risk—the same is true for ecstatic relationships. The Resilient Edge of Resistance of a relationship is maintained by change.

S. Bear Bergman, quoted in Tristan Taormino's book *Opening Up* offers some wise advice:

> "Let your relationships be what they are. Relationships seem to have their own trajectories, their own needs and wants and expiration dates, their own purposes. Being open to how relationships grow and shift is very difficult and very necessary. Sometimes a friend becomes a lover, a lover becomes a friend, sometimes the right person appears at exactly the right time for a specific purpose. (And when that purpose is done, sometimes disappears entirely . . .) Sometimes the perfect relationship to have with someone is an extravagant dinner and delicious sex—twice a year. Even if they live around the corner."

It is necessary for some relationships to end in order for other relationships to begin, or for other opportunities in your life to unfold.

My friend Lolita Wolf said something wise and healing when I was grieving the loss of a relationship. Lolita asked, "Did you have a profound connection—unlike anything you'd ever had before? Did you go to amazing places together, create outrageous adventures, and have incredible sex? Do you feel like you're a much bigger and better person for having been in this relationship?" "Yes," I said through my tears. "In that case," said Lolita, "congratulations on such a successful relationship."

Ecstatic Emotional and Spiritual Practices

Many of the emotional and spiritual practices we discussed in the closing circle of the Australian Urban Tantra Professional Training Program were activities that might be part of any daily spiritual practice, and many of them have been described—either in passing or in depth—in our explorations of the many possible paths to ecstasy.

A few of the practices, however, seemed particularly pertinent to the process of living an ecstatic life with an emphasis on the erotic. I offer them here in the form of affirmations for you to interpret in your own way.

- I embrace my authentic feelings.

- I love fiercely.

- I am willing to drop my armor and expose my vulnerabilities.

- I am ready to release old wounds.

- I know when to leap forward, and when to stop.

- I am willing to stretch my boundaries.

- I say yes to everything.

- I see beauty in every mundane moment.

- I am consistently present at ever-deepening levels in each moment.

- It's okay to run away.

- It's okay to just be.

- I create my universe day by day.

- I am living my ecstasy right now.

The Ecstatic Life Playsheet

This playsheet will help you to launch and maintain your ecstatic life practice. You can make photocopies and fill out a new playsheet whenever you feel the need to check in—or to see where you might like to go next—in the process of your ecstatic and erotic evolution.

My Ecstatic Life Playsheet

My top ten turn-ons in life are:

1.

2.

3.

4.

5.

6.

7.

8.

9.

10.

My favorite sexual activity to receive is:

My favorite sexual activity to give is:

My favorite place in nature is:

My favorite physical pleasure is:

The one (or more) thing(s) that always bring(s) me more deeply into my body is/are:

The one (or more) thing(s) that always make(s) me feel like I am flying is/are:

My favorite way to connect with other people is:

The spiritual practice that best supports my ecstatic life is:

AFTERCARE

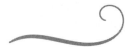

After an orgasm or an ecstatic experience, you are in a powerful trance state—it's quite possibly the most important and powerful time in any ecstatic ritual. In Tantra, the period of time following lovemaking is often called the afterglow. In BDSM, there is a practice called aftercare. Just as its name implies—aftercare is what happens in the afterglow immediately following a BDSM scene. In the stillness that follows intense erotic activity people may very well experience the most meaningful part of their journey. Some people see colors or visions; some hear music or a universal hum; others feel waves of emotion. Some people feel a deeper intimacy with their partner; others may feel an intimacy with all of creation.

It is crucial to support someone with care and mindfulness while they are in this state. Even after your partner appears to be regaining something resembling ordinary consciousness, they are still in a fragile and receptive state. It's important to be closely attentive to someone in this state, and to treat them with love and consciousness. They may want a glass of water, or a cup of tea, or hot cocoa. They may need to be kept warm, or they may need to cool down under running water. Offer them something to eat. Cuddle them in a blanket in your arms. Or walk them outside and lie them down under the stars. Stay with them until they can tell you that they feel like they're back in their body and that they are beginning to integrate the ecstatic experience. And just as important: ask for this kind of care for yourself, should you be the one who winds up in the blaze or the hush of afterglow.

Remember, inner transformation can continue long after you've both stopped playing. Either you or both of you may have a revelation a week later. Waves of released emotion may wash over either of you 24 or 48 hours later. You may need or want to talk to the person or people who accompanied you on the journey. Unless otherwise negotiated, it is customary for two (or more) people to agree that they can contact each other for further support.

In this spirit, as we end our journey through this guide to ecstasy, I'd like to bring you a symbolic cup of cocoa—or glass of champagne, if you prefer. I'd like to hold you close and say:

> Well done, you! You have been so courageous and so delightful to play with. I have loved every moment I have spent exploring ecstasy with you, and I hope you've found something valuable along the way. Thank you for trusting me and for letting me into your inner life.

> I'd like to continue the journey with you. Please join me at a workshop, on Facebook (BarbaraCarrellasUrbanTantra), or on Twitter (urbantantrika).

> Until our paths cross again, I wish you an ecstatic journey.

> Ecstatically yours,

Barbara

www.BarbaraCarrellas.com

Afterglow A

Sexual Pain: Common Symptoms, Causes, and Treatments

I want to take a moment and talk about some of the causes of pain during sex in the hope that providing this information will lead to more discussion and treatment.

For women (or people of any gender with vaginas and vulvas), one of the most common causes of vaginal pain is dryness. This kind of pain happens at the vaginal opening, right at the beginning of any kind of vaginal penetration. Lack of natural lubrication might be due to changes in hormone levels at certain times in the menstrual cycle, lower estrogen levels after menopause, or while breast-feeding, or not being sufficiently aroused. And some women just don't produce as much natural lubrication as others. A water-based lubricant can make all the difference. Water-based lubes come in all sorts of varieties, from flavored to organic. They are preferable to oil-based lubes (including lube alternatives such as baby oil, Vaseline, and lotion) because water-based lubes won't damage condoms, and the body can flush them out much more easily. If your lack of lubrication is simply because you aren't turned on enough for your body to make its own lubrication, then spend more time in the arousal phase of sex prior to penetration. However, I recommend having plenty of lube on hand in any case. If you're looking for the kind of prolonged sexual encounters that lead to ecstatic experiences you'll want lube on hand in order to stay slippery and comfortable.

Another source of pain for women might be inflammation of the tissue of the vulva. The inflammation might be caused by a yeast infection, genital warts, herpes, or an infected benign cyst (called a Bartholin's gland cyst). If you are experiencing burning, soreness, a thick whitish discharge, fleshy raised bumps, itching, tingling, ulcers, pain or swelling of the labia, see your doctor.

Vaginismus is a condition in which the muscles around the opening of the vagina spasm shut. Spasms like these can make penetration feel painful, burning, uncomfortable, or unachievable. Continued attempts at penetration create further discomfort. Here's why:

When the body anticipates pain, it automatically tightens the vaginal muscles, which reinforces the reflex response, creating a cycle of pain. The root causes of vaginismus usually have a strong emotional component. Vaginismus is highly treatable with a combination of pelvic floor exercises, gradual dilation, techniques to reduce pain, and exercises designed to help women identify, express, and resolve any contributing emotional components. Check out www.vaginismus.com for more information and resources.

Other types of pain that happen right at the beginning of any kind of vaginal penetration can be caused by scars from an episiotomy (an incision made in the tissue between the vaginal opening and perineum during childbirth). Vaginal infections such as cystitis (inflammation of the bladder) can cause burning pain, a strong persistent urge to urinate, and lower abdominal pain.

The cause of an occasional *deeper* pain for women during intercourse may be as simple as a change in the position of the cervix that happens over the course of a month. But there are other possible causes, such as fibroids, endometriosis, ovarian cysts, and pelvic inflammatory disease. See your doctor if you are experiencing any intense deep pain, or if you experience deep pain on a regular basis.

The most common types of sexual pain for men are pain during or after ejaculation, and testicular pain. Pain after ejaculation can be caused by prostatitis, an inflammation or infection of the prostate gland that can cause swelling and pain in the penis and testicles, or in the perineum (the area between the scrotum and anus). Prostatitis can also cause pain during ejaculation. Epididymitis, a swelling of the tube that connects the testicle with the vas deferens, can also cause a tender, swollen groin and pain during ejaculation.

Peyronie's disease is one of the more common causes of sexual pain in men. The characteristic sign is a visible curvature or hourglass shape of the penis when erect. Physical damage to the penis—which can be caused by minor trauma to the penis during sex, or as a result of a sports injury—results in the formation of scar tissue. The section of the sheath with scar tissue is no longer flexible. Therefore, when the penis becomes erect, the region with the scar tissue doesn't stretch, and the penis bends or becomes disfigured. Peyronie's disease is essentially arthritis of the penis and it can be very painful. It is often treated with arthritis medication, steroids, injections, and in the most severe cases, surgery.

Other causes of sexual pain in men are urinary tract infections, yeast infections, psoriasis, and dermatitis, the latter of which can be caused by an allergy to chemicals or soaps. If you are experiencing a strong persistent urge to urinate or burning pain when urinating, lower abdominal pain, itching, burning at the tip of your penis, a rash or scaly skin on your penis or scrotum, see your doctor.

Painful conditions specifically related to uncircumcised men include phimosis, a condition in which the foreskin is too tight to be completely retracted over the head of the penis, and paraphimosis, a condition in which the foreskin is stuck behind the head of the penis and can't be pulled forward.

Sexually transmitted diseases such as chlamydia, genital warts, gonorrhea, hepatitis, herpes, HIV, molluscum contagiosum (aka MC or water warts), scabies, syphilis, thrush, and trichomoniasis are just a few of the sexually transmitted diseases that can cause pain in people of all genders.

The first step in alleviating any physical pain during sex is to determine if there is a body-level cause that needs help or treatment. And yes, pain during sex may simply be a sign that you need to slow down and use more lube. However, any occurrence of sexual pain that is not easily alleviated by one or both of these methods should be taken seriously and investigated by a medical professional.

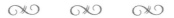

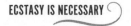

Afterglow B

Safer-Sex Guidelines

Remember: The time to make safer-sex decisions is before you take your clothes off. Everyone should have a basic safe-sex supply kit within easy reach. You don't need a lot of stuff to play safely. You can put a safer-sex kit together with a few essential basics.

Condoms

Use latex condoms for all intercourse—vaginal or anal. They help protect against gonorrhea, syphilis, chlamydia, herpes, hepatitis B, and AIDS. Use condoms on your sex toys, if you use them with others. They work on dildos, anal plugs, and vibrators. Use a new condom for each partner who uses the toy. Never reuse a condom.

For oral sex, use an unlubricated or flavored condom. A word of warning—condoms lubricated with Nonoxynol-9 taste terrible! You can also cut a condom lengthwise, open it up, and place it over the anus or vulva for oral-anal sex (rimming) or oral-vaginal sex (cunnilingus).

Lube

Use plenty of water-based lube on the outside of the condom for comfort, mutual pleasure, and to keep the condom from tearing during sex. Some men find that more sensation is transmitted to them if they put a small amount of water-based or silicone-based lube inside the tip of their condom before putting it on. Use only water-based or silicone lubricants on condoms. Oil-based lubricants, such as Vaseline, Crisco, and hand lotions, weaken latex and make condoms break.

Gloves

Do you need to wear gloves before you touch someone's genitals or anus? Here's a test: Cut a lemon in half and rub it all over your hands and fingers. (Vinegar or alcohol-based hand sanitizer works as well as lemons.) If you feel any stinging, you have breaks in your skin that could let germs enter or exit your bloodstream. Glove up! You can buy latex, vinyl, or nitrile gloves at a drugstore or medical supply store. If you want to do anal play with an oil-based lube (which some people prefer), be sure to get vinyl or nitrile gloves. Vinyl and nitrile are not compromised by oil the way latex is.

Plastic wrap

Plain old plastic food wrap is the best barrier for rimming and cunnilingus. Do not use the type specifically advertised for microwave ovens, as it has little holes in it that defeat the purpose of a barrier. You can roll out a piece of plastic wrap large enough to cover both vulva and anus. It's much easier to hang onto than a cut-open condom, and it's a lot thinner than a dental dam. Spread some lube on your partner's side of the plastic wrap for increased sensation. Just make sure that the plastic wrap doesn't touch the anus and then the vulva. Germs passed from anus to vagina can cause a nasty infection.

Some people do prefer dental dams for oral sex, but I find them too thick and too hard to hold on to. It's easy to drop a dam when it gets slippery, and then you may not be able to tell which side has been against the body.

A Note About Oral Sex: Some people feel that safer-sex barriers are not as necessary for oral sex as they are for vaginal and anal sex. I disagree. Yes, it's clear that the risk of transmitting HIV is much lower for unprotected oral sex than for unprotected anal or vaginal intercourse. But this is not true for transmission of herpes, gonorrhea, syphilis, and chlamydia. And the risk of transmitting all these STIs is greater if you have any open sores in your mouth, or periodontal disease.

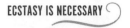

The Female Condom

The female condom is a plastic sheath that women can insert in their vaginas for use in protection against HIV and STIs. The female condom can be inserted up to eight hours before sex, has rings at both ends to hold it in place, and can be lubricated with oil-based lubricants that stay wet longer than the water-based variety. This kind of condom takes practice to use, and it's more expensive than a latex condom. Some people also use the female condom for anal sex. Although it has not been officially approved for this use, many people find them very effective.

Special Situations

The following situations present special issues relating to safer sex and require customized safer-sex kits. Customize your kit accordingly.

Water Sports

It's safe to urinate on skin without open cuts or sores. Use the lemon/vinegar test. Urine that enters the mouth, vagina, or rectum is not safe. It could spread HIV or hepatitis B.

Blood Sports

Serious aficionados of piercings, cuttings, or any kind of blood sports know that the lighting has to be bright, the instruments sterile, and the protocol impeccable to keep everyone safe. Any of these more arcane pleasure techniques, done incorrectly, could result in permanent injury or transmission of serious disease. You'll need to learn both the techniques and the hygienic protocol from an experienced person. Merely seeing it done once or twice is not enough! Ask an experienced player to teach you how to do things safely and with maximum pleasure, and exactly what you'll need to add to your safer-sex kit.

A Note about Hepatitis A, B, C

Hepatitis is an umbrella term for seven types of viral infections that cause inflammation of the liver. Hepatitis A, B, and C are the most common types. Many people do not think of hepatitis as a sexually transmitted disease, but in reality, all three common strains of hepatitis can be passed on through various types of sexual contact. Each strain has different causes and symptoms. It's important to understand the properties of each so you can plan your safer-sex protocol accordingly.

Hepatitis A is spread through contact with the feces of an infected person. Hepatitis A infection can begin when only the tiniest amount of feces gets inside another person's mouth. It can be passed on sexually, particularly during activities such as anilingus (oral-anal sex, a.k.a. rimming). Washing of genital and anal areas before sex, combined with the use of condoms, dental dams, or plastic wrap can help to significantly lower this risk. Hepatitis A can be prevented by immunization. There is no specific treatment for hepatitis A. Most people fight off the virus naturally, returning to full health within a couple of months.

Hepatitis B is similar to hepatitis A in its symptoms, but is more likely to cause chronic long-term illness and permanent damage to the liver if not treated. Hepatitis B is most frequently passed on through the exchange of bodily fluids with an infected person. Hepatitis B is estimated to be 50 to 100 times more infectious than HIV. All safer-sex precautions are recommended.

Hepatitis B can be prevented by immunization. There is no specific treatment, and as with hepatitis A, most patients recover on their own in a few months. In approximately 5 percent of adult cases (and a much higher percentage in children and infants) hepatitis B infection will become chronic.

The hepatitis C virus is transferred through blood, and is more persistent than hepatitis A or B. It is ten times more infectious than HIV and four to five times more prevalent. Hepatitis C causes liver damage that can result in cirrhosis and cancer. Treatments have improved but are only 50 percent effective. Hepatitis C cannot be passed on by hugging, sneezing, coughing, sharing food or water, sharing cutlery, or casual contact. It can only be contracted through exposure to the blood of an infected person through unprotected sex (if blood is present because of genital sores, cuts or menstruation) or through erotic blood sports such as piercing, cutting, or tattooing.

Currently, there is no vaccine for hepatitis C, and treatments combining the antiviral drugs interferon and ribavirin are only 50 percent effective. The antiviral drugs may cause significant side effects that may be intolerable for some people.

You greatly reduce your chances of contracting any strain of hepatitis when you practice safer sex. So please, get tested. Ask your partners to get tested. And take appropriate precautions.

Remember: While practicing safer sex dramatically reduces the risk of contracting or passing on the most serious sexually transmitted ailments, it does not completely eliminate the risk for every possible condition.

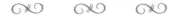

Afterglow C

Non-Monogamy, Open-Relationship, and Polyamory Resources

(Listed in alphabetical order)

Books:

The Ethical Slut, by Dossie Easton and Janet W. Hardy

Love In Abundance: A Counselor's Advice on Open Relationships, by Kathy Labriola

Opening Up, by Tristan Taormino

Pagan Polyamory, by Raven Kaldera

Polyamory: The New Love Without Limits, by Deborah Anapol

Polyamory: Roadmaps for the Clueless & Hopeful by Anthony D. Ravenscroft

Redefining Our Relationships: Guidelines for Responsible Open Relationships by Wendy-O Matik

Internet Resources:

FetLife. www.fetlife.com is a free social network for the BDSM and fetish community. It's similar to Facebook and MySpace but run by kinky people. There are dozens of groups you can join that feature intelligent, thoughtful, and provocative discussions on polyamory and other styles of non-monogamy.

Franklin's Poly Pages. www.xeromag.com/fvpoly.html. This site is widely regarded as a most authoritative set of online advice on polyamory. It takes a fun and pragmatic tone and covers subjects

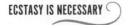

that are not as well-covered in the books, like mono/poly relationships and being a secondary.

Freaksexual. freaksexual.wordpress.com. Freaksexual is a wonderful blog in which Pepper deals intelligently and accessibly with issues surrounding polyamory and sexuality. The entries are more essays than posts. They're excellent reading regardless of how well acquainted you are with polyamory, but they're particularly valuable if you're just starting out.

OkCupid. www.okcupid.com. This free personals site has a very strong matching system and a kink-friendly and bi-friendly approach. This is not specifically a polyamory or non-monogamy site, but the matching is flexible and as a result, if you are non-monogamous, your top matches will share your style.

Polymatchmaker. www.polymatchmaker.com. This is the premier polyamory-specific personals site, with a good set of discussion forums and a strong mix of members, including queer folks and couples.

PolyWeekly Podcast. www.polyweekly.com. These are a series of half-hour radio-show–style segments on polyamory. They can be downloaded or streamed. The host, Minx, is charming and engaging, and the audio format allows her to cover a lot of territory. Most of the shows are on polyamory how-to subjects, but she also mixes in interviews and erotica readings.

Practical Polyamory. www.practicalpolyamory.com. This is the website of polyamory skills educator and advocate, Anita Wagner. This site is a great poly resource center. It features polyamory programs, a blog, downloadable documents, media resources, and referrals to poly-friendly therapists.

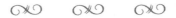

Afterglow D

How To Have A Breath and Energy Orgasm

Lie comfortably on your back, with your knees up, and your feet flat on the floor. Keep your spine straight. Don't use a pillow.

Relax your jaw. Yawn. Feel the back of your throat open.

Breathe in and out through your mouth—or, if it feels more comfortable—breathe in through your nose and exhale through your mouth. The important thing is to take in as much air as possible in a relaxed manner.

Think of your breath as a circle, with no pause between the inhale and the exhale. Don't force the exhale. If you make a little sighing sound on the exhale, you'll hear that you're not pushing too hard.

As you inhale, let your belly fill up like a balloon. As you exhale, flatten your lower back to the ground. This rocking motion helps to move sexual energy.

Add PC Squeezes. Most people like to squeeze on the exhale, but do what feels right for you.

Use your breath and your imagination to pull energy into your perineum (the area between your genitals and your anus, also known as the root chakra.) If it helps, you can drop a long, imaginary, taproot from your perineum down into an infinite source of red-hot energy at the center of the earth. Energy easily follows thought—you do not have to force it. All you have to do is focus on each area into which you are breathing and the energy will follow. You may find it helpful to place your hands on your body at each chakra point as you breathe into it.

Now, breathe your energy up to the sex center (lower belly, at the second chakra). Continue until your sex center feels charged up, lit up, bigger, or more alive. Trust yourself; you'll know when it is charged. You will feel that you're ready to move on, or it will feel as if the energy is moving up by itself.

241

If at any point you aren't feeling much (or nothing at all) just keep breathing. Fake it until you *do* feel it.

Now, breathe the energy up into your solar plexus (third chakra). It's located just below your diaphragm. Keep rocking and doing your PC squeezes. Continue until this area is well charged up.

Keep breathing! By now you may (or may not) be feeling some of the physical or emotional effects of the breath and energy orgasm.

Next, breathe the energy up into your heart center (fourth chakra). After this area is charged, breathe the energy up into your throat (fifth chakra). By the time the energy reaches your throat, you'll probably want to make some sounds. If sighs or sounds haven't happened naturally yet, it's important to vocalize them at this point. It will help build the energy.

By now, the energy may or may not be moving up your body on its own. If it is, just keep breathing and enjoy the experience. If the energy does not feel like it's moving on its own, intentionally breathe it up into the third eye (the middle of your forehead—the sixth chakra). Roll your eyes up (closed) as though you can see out the top of your head; it will help the energy rise.

The last chakra is the seventh, at the crown, just above the top of your head.

Remember: By the time you reach these higher chakras, the energy will most likely be flowing on its own. Just keep breathing and you will feel yourself moving rapidly into an orgasmic state.

Helpful Hints

If at any point in the process you feel that you have lost the plot and aren't feeling anything, don't get discouraged, and don't think you're doing something wrong. Energy levels may rise and fall. Just return to the area where the energy seems to have settled and start again from there. Or, go all the way back to the root chakra and pull energy from there directly into whichever higher chakra you're trying to energize.

Stay focused by using your hands to touch the chakras you're breathing into. Or, move your hands in small circles, as if lifting the energy up with each inhalation.

Raise the pitch of your voice on your exhalations as you move the energy up each chakra. This is particularly true as you circle energy in the higher chakras.

Do not be alarmed if you experience lightheadedness, dizziness, or tingling sensations or spasms and constrictions in your hands and feet. These effects are harmless and temporary. Take slow, deep breaths. The symptoms should pass in a short time. If you experience these symptoms, it may mean you are trying too hard. Ease up!

The Clench and Hold

Here's an additional breath and energy orgasm technique. You can add it to the technique above—after you have breathed the energy up into the top of your head. Or you can use it separately, anytime you have charged yourself up with breath.

When you're ready to do the Clench and Hold, take 30 or so fuller, faster breaths to really boost the energy.

Lie with your legs flat on the floor.

Take a full, deep breath. Fill up your lungs from bottom to top. Then let it all go without forcing your breath out.

Take another full, deep breath. Let it go, gently and fully.

Take a third deep breath. Fill up with as much air as you can hold . . . and . . . hold that breath!

Now here's the important part: As you're holding in your third breath, tense up every muscle in your body, especially your abdominal muscles, your butt muscles, and your PC muscle. It won't matter much if your hands or your feet aren't clenched, but if your abs, butt, and PC muscle aren't clenched, the Clench and Hold won't be as effective.

There are a number of ways to do this clench:

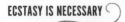

- Press down into the floor with your hands and shoulders and head and butt and legs and feet.

- Alternatively, extend your body as far as it can go; reach for the opposite wall with your feet and with your hands.

- Or, pull in toward the center of your body as hard as you can; first clench your abs, then pull the rest of your body in toward your abs.

However you do it, make sure you don't bring your knees up toward your stomach. This releases your abdominal muscles, and that's exactly what you don't want to do!

Keep tensing for about 15 seconds, then let go.

Now, here is the hardest part of the Clench and Hold for most people: Have no expectations. Don't try to make anything happen. You have given yourself a huge gift of openness and energy. Just be.

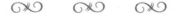

ACKNOWLEDGMENTS

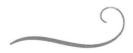

I first envisioned this book with inspiration and encouragement from Dossie Easton, who shares my passion for—and fascination with—the ecstatic experience. Essential new insights were revealed in the food court of The Maine Mall (and beyond) thanks to Dr. Mona Lisa Schulz. Its final shape and voice emerged under the elegant nurturance of my extraordinary editor, Patricia Gift.

Cheryl Richardson and I became friends during the writing of this book. I am deeply grateful to her for her enthusiasm for my work and for her invaluable feedback at so many crucial moments.

Huge thanks to David Houston, who read a late draft and offered important insights and suggestions. Thanks also to Laura Koch and Sally Mason at Hay House, and to my research assistant, Nick Foos. Very special thanks to my personal assistant, Jasmine Goldman, whose contributions on behalf of this book continue to be invaluable.

Gobs of gratitude to Barry R. Komisaruk and Nan Wise of Rutgers University, and David Erickson and Michele Spinak of Sirens Media for their patience and good humor in helping me to discover the brain science behind breath and energy orgasms. Special thanks to Sarah Sloane for her support in the process.

Acres of appreciation to Fakir Musafar, Grin Grindatti, Neo

Collette, Seth Cameron, Sharrin Spector, and Pat Baile for inspiring and nurturing me throughout the branding workshop.

My sisters of the heart and co-conspirators in erotic education and enlightenment—Annie Sprinkle, Hayley Caspers, Catherine Carter, Cyndi Darnell and Liana Gailand—have consistently contributed to my work, my life, and to this book in profound and delightful ways. I love you all deeply.

I couldn't do what I do, be who I am, or know what I know without the love and support of a legion of stellar friends and colleagues. These co-conspirators made significant contributions to this book: Corey Alexander, Phoenix Benner, S. Bear Bergman, Justin Vivian Bond, Seema Chandarana, Avika deVine, Ullie Emigh, Femcar, Amy Jo Goddard, Janet Hardy, Lin Hill, Patricia Johnson, Jwala, Joseph Kramer, Maya Labos, Denise Linn, Wendy-O Matik, Mark Michaels, Reid Mihalko, Marilyn S. Miller, Casey Morgan, Judith Orloff, M.D., Marcelle Pick, Donna Poulin, Carl Johan Rehbinder, Tristan Taormino, Tessa Wills, and Lolita Wolf.

The final chapter, *Living an Ecstatic Life,* was co-created with the participants of the first graduating class of the Australian Urban Tantra® Professional Training Program. Thank you, dear colleagues: Alex Rossiter, Ally, Ambrosia, Breanna Sheets, Cate Jones, Cyd Saunders, Danniel Shervey, Deej Juventin, Electra A'more, Irene, Jack Lee Adams, Janine McDonald, Kirsteen A Farley, Lady Ambrosia, Oscar Gettar, Phillip C Gordon, Scarlett Wallingford, Silverback11, Suzie Donkin, Uma Furman.

My deepest gratitude to the members of my Facebook and Twitter focus group who contributed so eloquently to the totality of ecstatic possibilities: Alfred Surillo, Anita Wagner, Betty Devoe, Betty Herbert, Betty Martin, Bill Slette, Bootie Berry, Brian Gleason, Brian Hammond, Candye Kane, Charos, Chrissy Cologne, Christina Bjornelf, Christopher Stewart, Dan Middleton, David Franklin Farkas, David Wilkins, Diana Jaramillo, Diane Ray DePasquale, DK Daddy, Dominique Kalata, Donia Love, Enterblisstonia, Eric Wunderman, Eve Katz, Gary Lynn Tucker, Hector Aguilar, Ingrid Geronimo, Joanne Morton, Katherine Matthews, Kathryn

Smith, Katie Sarra, Kelly Webb, Ken Ng, Lesley B. Alexander, Lisa Vandever, Lubyanka, Lynn Paterson, Marina Fick, Meg Barker, Meir Calloway, Mette Welhaven Naess, Nancy L. Hill, Neon Wiess, Olivia Jade, Pete Stone, Philip Coupal, Philip Jean-Pierre, Rick Umbaugh, Rodney DeJong, Roger Gindi, Rory Brennan, Rowan Tinca Parkes, Sara Denward, Shelley Anderson, Siri Chand Singh, Soleil Feliz, Sylvia Machatt, Tim Doody, Todd Kamensky, Tyr Throne, Vera Worthington, Vincent Hewett, Viviane Tang, Wes Wolcott, and Zee McClelland.

Thanks also to my clients, workshop participants and to the callers to my Hay House Radio show who provided stories, wisdom, and countless displays of courage.

I am thrilled and delighted to be working in this new capacity with my friends and family at Hay House. Humongous hunks of gratitude to you all, especially Reid Tracy, Margarete Nielsen, Nancy Levin, Gail Gonzales, Donna Abate, and Christy Salinas.

Deep and ongoing thanks to my agent, Malaga Baldi, who regularly provides me with inspiration and encouragement as well as sound business advice.

I am tingling with delight—for a second time (the first was *Urban Tantra*)—over the ecstatic cover art designed by Kate Basart of Union Pageworks.

Bless you, Karen Bell, for the mala, and Buc Horyn, for including me in the Santa Barbara ritual and for the gifts from the beach. These mattered more than you know.

This book would not have happened without the unconditional love and inspiration of my loved ones, especially:

Chester Mainard: Even in nonphysical you continue to provoke the best in me. It continues to be a delight to co-create with you. Thank you for showing up at all the right times.

The four-leggeds—PKitty, Mollyanna, Calla Lily, Maui, Gizmo and Bruce—each of you plays an invaluable role in keeping me on purpose and in my body. Scritches, rubs, and bonks to you all.

Louise L. Hay: Thank you for your generosity, your passion, your wild spirit, your uncompromising honesty, and your

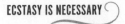

unrelenting belief in me. Thank you for 25 years of unconditional love. I adore you.

And Kate Bornstein, my partner in life, love, and art: Thank you for reading and editing every page of this book—especially while you were in the midst of writing your own. Your love, encouragement, and support of my ecstatic pursuits—however weird and wild—have made all the difference. I love and treasure you, Imzadi.

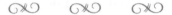

ABOUT THE AUTHOR

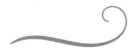

Barbara Carrellas is an author, sex educator, sex/life coach, university lecturer, workshop facilitator, motivational speaker, and theatre artist. Her most recent books are *Urban Tantra: Sacred Sex for the Twenty-First Century* and *Luxurious Loving.* Barbara's pioneering Urban Tantra® workshops were named best in New York City by *Time Out New York* magazine. She is the co-founder of Erotic Awakening, a groundbreaking series of workshops that toured the United States and Australia. She has also written and produced *The Pleasure Principle,* an educational audio series.

As a sex/life coach, Barbara offers her clients a practical, intuitive, and informative approach to realizing their deepest desires. The essence of all of her work is the inseparable connection between one's sex life and the rest of one's life, and the happy integration of body, mind, and spirit.

Barbara has lectured at many educational institutions, including Harvard University, Brown University, Vassar College, Dartmouth College, and Yale University. She is a popular keynote speaker and presents workshops internationally on sex and spirituality.

Barbara is a certified sexologist (ACS, American College of Sexologists) and a member of AASECT (American Association of Sexuality Educators, Counselors and Therapists). She is also a proud graduate of the Coney Island Sideshow School with a double major in fire eating and snake handling.

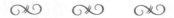

Hay House Titles of Related Interest

YOU CAN HEAL YOUR LIFE, *the movie,*
starring Louise L. Hay & Friends
(available as a 1-DVD program and an expanded 2-DVD set)
Watch the trailer at: **www.LouiseHayMovie.com**

THE SHIFT, *the movie,*
starring Dr. Wayne W. Dyer
(available as a 1-DVD program and an expanded 2-DVD set)
Watch the trailer at: **www.DyerMovie.com**

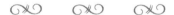

THE ART OF EXTREME SELF-CARE: *Transform Your Life One
Month at a Time,* by Cheryl Richardson

LOVE YOUR BODY, by Louise L. Hay

SECRETS OF ATTRACTION: *The Universal Laws of Love, Sex,
and Romance,* by Sandra Anne Taylor

THE TOTALITY OF POSSIBILITIES, by Louise L. Hay

All of the above are available at your local bookstore,
or may be ordered by contacting Hay House (see next page).

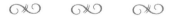

We hope you enjoyed this Hay House book. If you'd like to receive our online catalog featuring additional information on Hay House books and products, or if you'd like to find out more about the Hay Foundation, please contact:

Hay House, Inc., P.O. Box 5100, Carlsbad, CA 92018-5100
(760) 431-7695 or (800) 654-5126
(760) 431-6948 (fax) or (800) 650-5115 (fax)
www.hayhouse.com® • **www.hayfoundation.org**

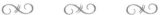

Published and distributed in Australia by: Hay House Australia Pty. Ltd., 18/36 Ralph St., Alexandria NSW 2015 • *Phone:* 612-9669-4299 • *Fax:* 612-9669-4144 www.hayhouse.com.au

Published and distributed in the United Kingdom by: Hay House UK, Ltd., 292B Kensal Rd., London W10 5BE • *Phone:* 44-20-8962-1230 • *Fax:* 44-20-8962-1239 www.hayhouse.co.uk

Published and distributed in the Republic of South Africa by: Hay House SA (Pty), Ltd., P.O. Box 990, Witkoppen 2068 • *Phone/Fax:* 27-11-467-8904 www.hayhouse.co.za

Published in India by: Hay House Publishers India, Muskaan Complex, Plot No. 3, B-2, Vasant Kunj, New Delhi 110 070 • *Phone:* 91-11-4176-1620 *Fax:* 91-11-4176-1630 • www.hayhouse.co.in

Distributed in Canada by: Raincoast, 9050 Shaughnessy St., Vancouver, B.C. V6P 6E5 • *Phone:* (604) 323-7100 • *Fax:* (604) 323-2600 • www.raincoast.com

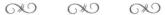

Take Your Soul on a Vacation

Visit **www.HealYourLife.com®** to regroup, recharge, and reconnect with your own magnificence. Featuring blogs, mind-body-spirit news, and life-changing wisdom from Louise Hay and friends.

Visit **www.HealYourLife.com** today!

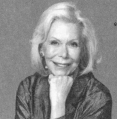
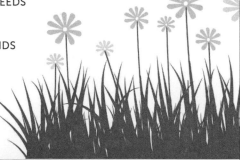